Eating and weight disorders

Carlos M. Grilo

Yale University School of Medicine

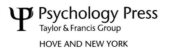

Psychology Press
Taylor & Francis Group

HOVE AND NEW YORK

First published 2006 by Psychology Press, part of Taylor and Francis
27 Church Road, Hove, East Sussex, BN3 2FA

Simultaneously published in the USA and Canada
by Psychology Press,
270 Madison Avenue, New York, NY 10016

Psychology Press is part of the Taylor and Francis Group, an informa business

Copyright © 2006 Psychology Press

Typeset in Palatino by Garfield Morgan, Mumbles, Swansea
Printed and bound in Great Britain by TJ International, Padstow, Cornwall
Cover design by Jim Wilkie

British Library Cataloguing in Publication Data
A catalogue record for this book is available from the British Library

Library of Congress Cataloging-in-Publication Data
Grilo, Carlos (Carlos M.)
    Eating disorders / Carlos Grilo.
        p. cam. – (Clinical psychology, a modular course)
    Includes bibliographical references and index.
    ISBN 13: (invalid) 978-1-84169-547-5 (hbk.)
    ISBN 13: (invalid) 978-1-84169-548-3 (pbk.)
    ISBN 10: 1-84169-547-5 (hbk.)
    ISBN 10: 1-84169-548-3 (pbk.)
    1. Eating disorders. I. Title. II. Series.
    RC552.E18G75 2006
    616.85'26–dc22

                                                    2005035699

    ISBN 13: 978-1-84169-547-5 hbk
    ISBN 13: 978-1-84169-548-3 pbk

    ISBN 10: 1-84169-547-5 hbk
    ISBN 10: 1-84169-548-3 pbk

Contents

Series preface

Clinical Psychology: A Modular Course was designed to overcome the problems faced by the traditional textbook in conveying what psychological disorders are really like. All the books in the series, written by leading scholars and practitioners in the field, can be read as stand-alone text, but they will also integrate with the other modules to form a comprehensive resource in clinical psychology. Students of psychology, medicine, nursing, and social work, as well as busy practitioners in many professions, often need an accessible but thorough introduction to how people experience anxiety, depression, addiction, or other disorders, how common they are, and who is most likely to suffer from them, as well as up-to-date research evidence on the causes and available treatments. The series will appeal to those who want to go deeper into the subject than the traditional textbook will allow, and base their examination answers, research projects, assignments, or practical decisions on a clearer and more rounded appreciation of the clinical and research evidence.

Chris R. Brewin

Other titles in this series:

Depression
Constance Hammen

Stress and Trauma
Patricia A. Resick

Childhood Disorders
Philip C. Kendall

Schizophrenia
Max Birchwood and Chris Jackson

Addictions
Maree Teesson, Louise Degenhardt and Wayne Hall

Anxiety
S. Rachman

Overview of eating and weight disorders
Bodies to die for

1

This book provides an overview of eating and weight disorders. Eating disorders refer to a range of problems characterized by abnormal eating behaviors and beliefs about eating, weight, and shape. Obesity refers to excess body fat. Most persons with eating disorders are not obese. Most obese persons do not have eating disorders although many may suffer from disordered eating. Eating and weight concerns appear to have become ubiquitous in westernized societies. A careful analysis by Colditz (1992) revealed that Americans spent roughly $33 billion annually in the early 1990s on a plethora of weight loss products and services. This spending on weight loss products grew to roughly $50 billion annually by the turn of the century. Eating and weight disorders are much more than just concerns with aesthetics. Eating disorders, which are classified as psychiatric problems, and obesity, which is classified as a general medical condition, reflect a diverse and perplexing array of biological, social, psychological phenomena.

As this book will summarize, eating and weight disorders reflect "bodies to die for" in many ways. At one end of the weight continuum is anorexia nervosa, a relatively rare problem affecting primarily young women. Individuals suffering from anorexia nervosa go to truly remarkable lengths to lose weight despite their emaciated states. Anorexia nervosa has one of the highest mortality rates of any psychiatric disorder (Sullivan, 1995) which translates to more than a twelve-fold increase in death rate relative to their age peers. At the other end of the weight continuum is obesity, a common problem that is continuing to increase in prevalence despite pervasive societal pressures and individual desires to achieve thinness. Obesity has one of the highest associated mortality rates of any medical condition. In the United States alone, over 300,000 premature deaths are attributable to obesity annually (Allison, Fontaine, Manson, Stevens, & VanItallie, 1999). Obesity substantially decreases life expectancy and increases early mortality (Peeters, Bonneux, Barendregt, &

Nusselder, 2003). The steady increase in life expectancy observed since the nineteenth century has slowed during the past three decades (Oeppen & Vaugel, 2002) and a recent sophisticated analysis suggests that the United States may face a decline in average life expectancy due to the effects of obesity on longevity (Olshansky et al., 2005).

In this introductory chapter, an overview of eating disorders and obesity is provided. Eating is an everyday behavior that addresses a very basic biological need for energy. Problems with eating and weight have undoubtedly always existed. There exist rich accounts of behaviors ranging from self-starvation (Vandereycken & Van Deth, 1994) to voracity and gorging (Parry-Jones & Parry-Jones, 1991; Stein & Laasko, 1988) dating back several centuries. Inspection of historical and medical sources, however, suggests that what we currently conceptualize as eating disorders may best be thought of as "new" or "modern" problems characteristic of the twentieth century (Vandereycken, 2002; Vandereycken & Van Deth, 1994). Similarly, obesity has likely always existed in civilized societies. Visitors to the western world's art museums readily recall the pervasive "plumpness" emphasized as the preferred or idealized body images throughout the fifteenth through eighteenth centuries. Bray (1993, 2002b), in his commentaries about early scientific contributions to energy balance and obesity, noted that a series of monographs appeared in the mid-nineteenth century including Banting's (1863) "A Letter on Corpulence Addressed to the Public" (reprinted as Banting (1993) Letter on corpulence addressed to the public, 3rd edition, in *Obesity Research*), which perhaps represents the first diet book.

Defining eating and weight disorders

Current classification or diagnostic schemes include eating disorders (abnormal eating behaviors and beliefs about eating and body shape) as psychiatric or mental disorders and obesity (excess body fat) as a general physical or medical condition. It can, at times, be difficult to determine what is aberrant or "non-normative" and how, or where, to draw a line. The major classification systems currently use categorical rather than dimensional methods to describe or label problems. Emerging research suggests that our conceptual models of eating-related problems are probably too simplistic and that neither categorical nor dimensional approaches adequately capture the full range of aberrant eating (Bulik, Sullivan, & Kendler, 2000a; Keel et al.,

2004; Williamson, Gleaves, & Stewart, 2005; Williamson et al., 2002). Categorical approaches, which reflect our evolving attempts to "carve nature at its joints," have both advantages and disadvantages, but nonetheless provide us with a common language or starting point.

Classification of eating disorders and obesity

Both of the major classification systems for psychiatric disorders, the *International Classification of Diseases, 10th revision* (ICD-10; World Health Organization [WHO], 1992) and the *Diagnostic and Statistical Manual of Mental Disorders, 4th edition* (DSM-IV; American Psychiatric Association [APA], 1994), include eating disorder diagnoses. At a general level, an eating disorder diagnosis – like any mental disorder category in the DSM-IV (APA, 1994) – refers to a clinically-meaningful behavioral or psychological pattern that is associated with distress (e.g., upsetting or painful symptoms) or disability (e.g., impairment in functioning) or with substantially increased risk of morbidity, disability, or mortality. Both DSM-IV and ICD-10 include two specific eating disorder diagnoses (Anorexia Nervosa and Bulimia Nervosa) and a general less-specified category (Eating Disorder Not Otherwise Specified in the DSM-IV or Atypical Eating Disorders in the ICD-10). Obesity is classified in the ICD-10 as a general medical condition but is not included in the DSM-IV because it has not been consistently associated with either a behavioral or a psychological pattern or syndrome. Note that if there is evidence that psychological features are salient and of importance in the cause or maintenance of an individual's obesity, this can be assigned a diagnosis of Psychological Factors Affecting Medical Condition.

There are also three disorders of feeding or eating (Pica, Rumination Disorder, and Feeding Disorder of Infancy or Early Childhood) included in a section labeled "Feeding and Eating Disorders of Infancy or Early Childhood" in the DSM-IV. These three childhood problems will not be considered in this book but are defined here for the reader. Pica refers to a persistent pattern of eating nonnutritive substances by young children. Rumination disorder refers to repeated regurgitation (without any observable nausea, disgust, or attempt to vomit) and rechewing of food without any gastrointestinal or medical reason. Feeding disorder of infancy or early childhood refers to the persistent failure to eat adequately and thus to gain sufficient weight for age.

TABLE 1.1

Anorexia nervosa: Definition and diagnostic criteria

A. Low weight (i.e., less than 85% of expected).
B. Intense fear of gaining weight or becoming fat.
C. Disturbance in perception, experience, or evaluation of weight or shape.
D. Amenorrhea in postmenarcheal females.

Specify subtype:
   Restricting type: not regularly engaged in binge eating or purging behaviors (self-induced vomiting or the misuse of laxatives, diuretics, or enemas).
   Binge eating/purging type: regularly engaged in binge eating or purging behaviors.

Based on the four criteria and subtyping in the *Diagnostic and statistical manual of mental disorders* (4th ed.; *DSM-IV*) published by the American Psychiatric Association (1994).

Anorexia nervosa (AN)

Table 1.1 lists the DSM-IV (APA, 1994) diagnostic criteria for anorexia nervosa. There are four criteria reflecting behavioral, psychological, and biological domains and there are two specified subtypes.

Refusal to maintain minimally normal weight

The first criterion, a behavioral criterion, is the refusal to maintain a minimally normal weight for age and height. This is defined as less than 85% of what is expected weight. This criterion can be met by a person losing weight to fall below 85% of what is normal or failing to gain weight during a period of growth or development and thus failing to achieve at least 85% of what is considered normal. There is general agreement about the need for this criterion although the exact weight threshold or optimal level is less clear. In principle it should clinically reflect when starvation symptoms take over or when physical problems or consequences begin. The ICD-10 includes a guideline of requiring a body mass index (kg/m^2) of less than 17.5.

In most cases, the low weight is achieved primarily by very severe or restrictive eating. Individuals typically begin by excluding or eliminating foods that are thought to be fattening resulting in reduced total food intake and weight loss. With increasing weight loss, the eating becomes increasingly restrictive in both quantity and type resulting in both greater weight loss and perceived control over food. Most individuals end up eating remarkably small and carefully selected amounts and types of (low fat) food. In addition to the very severe food restriction and periods of fasting, some individuals employ additional methods of weight loss including different purging methods (i.e., self-induced vomiting, misuse of laxatives or diuretics) and excessive exercise.

Intense fear of fat

The second criterion involves an intense fear of gaining weight or becoming fat. This fear can be rather intense and it is remarkable since the individual is, by any objective standard, considerably underweight. A common clinical observation is that this fear does not lessen with continued weight loss, but instead can actually intensify in many cases as the individual becomes even more emaciated. It is worth noting here that this criterion has evolved somewhat from earlier views that focused exclusively on the presumed body image disturbance driven primarily by overestimation of size. While many individuals with anorexia nervosa do substantially overestimate their size, this is not universal nor is it specific to anorexia nervosa. Current views highlight the attitudinal or psychological dimensions of these body concerns and intense fear of fatness.

Disturbance in perception, experience, or overevaluation of weight or shape

The third criterion, thought by many to represent the specific psychopathology of eating disorders, involves attitudinal and psychological disturbances in which weight and shape are experienced, weight and shape concerns unduly influence self-evaluation and self-worth, or a denial of the seriousness or danger of the low weight and extreme dieting. These specific disturbances distinguish eating disorders from other psychiatric problems.

Overall, this criterion can reflect a range in disturbance or distortion in how body weight and shape are experienced. Many individuals feel or experience their bodies globally as overweight while some have heightened and distressing concerns about specific body parts or regions. The ICD-10 focuses almost exclusively, and more narrowly than the DSM-IV, on this specific attitudinal disturbance (self-perception of being too fat and the fear or dread of fatness) as fueling the self-imposed low weight. Many individuals deny the seriousness of the low weight and its serious medical complications. Indeed, it is extraordinarily rare for an individual to voice concern about their weight loss even when it approaches truly dangerous levels.

The final example of this attitudinal disturbance involves the overevaluation of weight or shape. It is precisely this specific feature that is thought to represent the core psychopathology of eating disorders (Fairburn & Harrison, 2003). Individuals with eating disorders overevaluate their weight and shape and judge their self-esteem and self-worth primarily in terms of weight/shape and their ability to control them. Self-evaluation unduly influenced by weight/shape is a related but distinct feature from body dissatisfaction (Cooper & Fairburn, 1993; Masheb & Grilo, 2003). Body dissatisfaction is experienced by many individuals in our society regardless of whether or not they have an eating disorder. The ubiquitous nature of body shape concerns, particularly among women in westernized societies, has even been referred to as "normative discontent" (Rodin, Silberstein, & Striegel-Moore, 1985). The overevaluation criterion reflects a different concept. In contrast to most individuals who judge self-worth on the basis of several important aspects of their lives (e.g., relationships, roles as parents or partners, work or academic success, hobbies or activities, etc.), individuals with eating disorders tend to judge their self-worth based on their perception of their weight/eating and their perceived ability to control them.

Thus, in the case of an individual with anorexia nervosa, the weight loss and control over eating are viewed as important achievements. Not only is the weight loss not viewed as a problem, it is instead viewed as an important achievement or accomplishment. Similarly, the ability to severely restrict food intake is viewed as a sign of self-discipline and positive control. While this control continues it offers a slight boost to self-worth, but when perceived lapses in control occur significant emotional upset and distress follow. This core psychopathology explains the remarkable drive to control eating and weight and why these individuals have such limited motivation to follow suggestions to eat more.

Amenorrhea

The fourth criterion is, in postmenarcheal females, amenorrhea which is defined as the absence of at least three consecutive menstrual cycles. The amenorrhea is due to abnormally low levels of estrogen secretion and diminished secretion of follicle-stimulating hormone and luteinizing hormone by the pituitary. In prepubertal females, anorexia nervosa may delay menarche. Of note is that in the ICD-10 this criterion is referred to more broadly as a widespread endocrine disorder involving the hypothalamic-pituitary-gonadel axis, and lists loss of sexual interest and potency in men as an example in addition to the amenorrhea in women.

Amenorrhea in anorexia nervosa is poorly understood and is the target of considerable debate regarding its usefulness as a criterion (Cachelin & Maher, 1998). Amenorrhea is a common feature that seems to result, in part, from weight and body fat lost. Amenorrhea, however, is sometimes seen in individuals before large weight losses and sometimes persists after weight gain. Several studies have found that women with all of the features of anorexia nervosa except for amenorrhea do not differ from women with anorexia nervosa including amenorrhea (Garfinkel et al., 1996).

Subtypes of anorexia nervosa

DSM-IV specifies two subtypes of anorexia nervosa, "restricting type" and "binge-eating/purging type." The classification is based on the current pattern of symptoms. The majority of cases of anorexia nervosa are classified as "restricting type." Although evidence supports the distinction between these two subtypes of anorexia nervosa, as will be discussed further in chapter 2, it is not uncommon for individuals with anorexia nervosa to alternate between the restricting and the bingeing/purging subtypes at different points in their illness (Casper & Davis, 1977; Casper, Eckert, Halmi, Goldberg, & Davis, 1980; Eckert, Halmi, Marchi, Grove, & Crosby, 1995; Eddy, Keel, Dorer, Delinsky, Franko, & Herzog, 2002). A related but separate issue is that as many as 50% of patients with anorexia nervosa may eventually develop bulimia nervosa (Bulik, Sullivan, Fear, & Pickering, 1997b; Tozzi et al., 2005).

Restricting type

These individuals achieve their abnormally low weight by severely dieting, fasting, and often by exercising compulsively. Despite the seemingly frail or even emaciated physical state, some of these patients exhibit seemingly ceaseless activity and engage in high or even frenetic bouts of exercise (Davis et al., 1995, 1997). The extreme exercising behaviors seen in patients with anorexia nervosa frequently have a ritualistic or obsessive quality and are associated with higher levels of obsessive compulsiveness (Davis et al., 1995) and anxiety and somatization (Penas-lledo, Vaz Leal, & Waller, 2002).

Binge-eating/purging type

This subtype of anorexia nervosa is characterized by low weight and binge eating or purging through vomiting or misusing laxatives, enemas, or diuretics (these behaviors are described below). It is worth noting in the cases involving "binge eating," the amounts eaten are frequently not as large as seen (and required for meeting the binge eating criterion) in bulimia nervosa (described below). Research has found that the "binge-eating/purging type" differs from the "restricting type" in several ways, including greater likelihood of being overweight or having a family history of overweight, greater impulsivity, and higher rates of substance abuse (Casper et al., 1980; Garfinkel, Moldofsky, & Garner, 1980; Garfinkel, Kennedy, & Kaplan, 1995).

Bulimia nervosa (BN)

Table 1.2 lists the DSM-IV (APA, 1994) diagnostic criteria for bulimia nervosa and the two specified subtypes. It is important to begin by noting that the fifth criterion is that the person does not meet current criteria for anorexia nervosa. Thus, if an individual currently meets criteria for both anorexia nervosa and bulimia nervosa, the anorexia nervosa diagnosis is assigned. This hierarchy in the DSM-IV reflects the general consensus that anorexia is a more severe and chronic condition. Interestingly, in the ICD-10 the presence of certain features of bulimia nervosa (binge eating and a constant preoccupation or craving for food) precludes an individual from receiving a diagnosis of anorexia.

The criteria for bulimia nervosa have evolved from the seminal description provided by Russell (1979) in his paper entitled "Bulimia nervosa: An ominous variant of anorexia nervosa." This important paper, which quickly received support from studies in various countries (Abraham & Beumont, 1982; Fairburn & Cooper, 1982; Johnson, Stuckey, Lewis, & Schwartz, 1982; Pyle, Mitchell, & Eckert, 1981) stimulated considerable research on bulimia nervosa resulting in numerous important advances described later in this book. Although research since has highlighted many more differences between anorexia nervosa and bulimia nervosa than initially suggested by Russell (1979), the current criteria for purging type of bulimia nervosa correspond fairly well to his description, which included irresistible urges to overeat, compensatory behaviors, and the attitudinal feature of fear of fat.

TABLE 1.2

Bulimia nervosa: Definition and diagnostic criteria

A. Recurrent binge eating.
B. Recurrent inappropriate weight compensatory behaviors.
C. Binge eating and inappropriate weight compensatory behaviors both occur at least twice weekly over the past three months.
D. Overevaluation of weight and shape.
E. Does not meet criteria for anorexia nervosa.

Specify subtype:
   Purging type: regular use of self-induced vomiting or misuse of laxatives, diuretics, or enemas as the inappropriate weight compensatory method.
   Nonpurging type: regular use of fasting or excessive exercise as the inappropriate weight compensatory method but not regular use of the purging methods.

Based on the five criteria and subtyping in the *Diagnostic and statistical manual of mental disorders* (4th ed.; *DSM-IV*) published by the American Psychiatric Association (1994).

Recurrent binge eating

In the DSM-IV, bulimia nervosa is characterized behaviorally by recurrent episodes of binge eating and by recurrent inappropriate weight compensatory behaviors. The first criterion, binge eating, is defined as eating unusually large amounts of food (i.e., definitely larger than what most people would eat in the same context or under the same circumstances) in a discrete period of time (i.e., a two-hour period). In addition, the overeating episodes must occur while experiencing a clear sense of lack of control (i.e., inability to stop or control the eating). The DSM-IV also requires (third criterion for bulimia nervosa) that the binge eating occurs at least twice weekly over the past three months. A brief review of research on different aspects of binge eating follows.

What is the topography and nature of binge eating?

Early descriptions of binge eating among obese persons (Stunkard, 1959) and earlier versions of the DSM (i.e., the DSM-III-R published in 1987) defined binge eating as the rapid consumption of large amounts of food in a discrete period of time. Initial clinical descriptions also highlighted the emotional turmoil or distress during and after the eating (Stunkard, 1959) and stressed the irresistible nature of the urge to eat (Russell, 1979). Considerable research attempted to define the topography and nature of binge eating as it occurred naturally and in controlled laboratory settings (Walsh, Kissileff, & Hadigan, 1989).

This early research resulted in rich descriptive accounts and descriptions of binge eating that had both strengths and weaknesses. One strength of this early work is that it obtained information without, perhaps prematurely, imposing an arbitrary definition or preconceived set of criteria. One weakness was that the lack of a widely agreed upon definition of binge eating made it somewhat difficult to compare findings across studies. Nonetheless, inspection of the history of clinical and research studies suggests that while there is general consensus that the subjective sense of lack of control is the hallmark criterion for overeating to be labeled a binge, there is less agreement on what constitutes a "large amount."

Duration

Across diverse studies, patients' reports of their binge eating vary considerably. It appears that there is significant variability in the nature of binge eating *between* individuals as well as *within* individuals over time. In one of the first studies, Mitchell, Pyle, and Eckert (1981) obtained detailed reports of binge eating from 40 normal weight women with bulimia. In this patient group, the average duration of binge episodes was 1.18 hours with a range of 15 minutes to 8 hours. On average, these 40 patients spent roughly 13.7 hours per week engaging in binge eating, with a range of 30 minutes to 43 hours. Most subsequent clinical studies reported that most binge eating episodes are fairly discrete events that last less than one hour.

Frequency

The frequency of binge eating among patients with bulimia nervosa also varies considerably between individuals as well as within individuals over time. Mitchell and colleagues (1981), in their early study of 40 patients with bulimia, reported an average of 11.7 binges per week, with a range of 1 to 46 binges. Multiple daily binges are not uncommon in clinical samples of patients with bulimia. Fairburn and Cooper (1982), in another early study of 499 patients with bulimia, found that 27.2% of the participants reported binge eating on a daily basis. Other studies with clinical samples of bulimia have reported as many as 50% reporting daily binge episodes (Johnson et al., 1982; Pyle et al., 1981).

The variability in the frequency of binge eating did not point logically to an obvious cutpoint for determining a "clinically-meaningful" problem. The twice-weekly criterion adopted by the DSM-IV for establishing the diagnosis of bulimia nervosa is arbitrary. It was selected to prevent the diagnosis from being given to persons who infrequently binge (Wilson, 1992). Today, this requirement is followed by the majority of research studies. A recent treatment study for bulimia nervosa, which enrolled 220 patients, reported a median frequency of 6.25 binges per week (Agras, Walsh, Fairburn, Wilson, & Kraemer, 2000b). This frequency, which is typical for recent outpatient studies of bulimia nervosa, is lower than the early studies of patients with bulimia primarily due to the more rigorous current requirement that binge episodes must be unusually large. While this frequency of binge eating seems typical for clinical studies with treatment-seeking patients, there is reason to believe that patients with bulimia who do not seek treatment may differ somewhat (Fairburn, Welch, Norman, O'Connor, & Doll, 1996). The twice-weekly requirement has resulted in greater standardization in samples included in clinical and treatment studies but this practice may be excluding many patients who have clinically-meaningful problems. The few studies that have examined this issue have found no important differences in the clinical features of persons who binge at least once weekly versus twice or more weekly (Fairburn & Cooper, 1984; Garfinkel et al., 1995; Herzog, Hopkins, & Burns, 1993; Kendler et al., 1995; Wilson & Eldredge, 1991).

Food intake

In terms of food intake during binges, estimates based on quantities reported by patients using various different assessment methods vary considerably. There are isolated clinical reports of extreme examples or instances of food intake as high as 40,000 kcal (Abraham & Beumont, 1982; Hsu, 1990; Johnson & Connors, 1987). To put this figure in context, an intake of approximately 2000 kcal per day will result in fairly stable weight whereas 1200–1500 kcal/day is regarded as a moderate diet to result in a one pound weight loss per week. Perhaps more representative, Rosen, Leitenberg, Fisher, and Khazam (1986) estimated an average intake of 1459 kcal per binge for 199 binges reported by 20 females with bulimia during a one-week study period. Similar findings were reported by a study performed at Stanford University (Rossiter & Agras, 1990) in which 32 subjects with bulimia nervosa keep detailed food records (self-monitoring) for a week. During that week, the 32 patients had 343 binges that averaged roughly 1200 kcal per binge, although the range of intake during eating episodes was substantial. Of note, 28% of the eating episodes labeled as "binges" consisted of fewer than 500 kcal. Alternatively, other clinical and research reports noted that it was not uncommon for some individuals to eat large amounts of food without experiencing a loss or control or emotional upset. Such observations influenced diagnostic and research trends that emphasized the need to require both unusually large amount of food plus a clear subjective sense of loss of control as the working definition of a binge.

Considerable knowledge about eating disorders has also been gained from laboratory or "human-feeding" settings (Kaye, Weltzin, McKee, McConaha, Hansen, & Hsu, 1992). Naturalistic and clinical studies of eating disorders are potentially limited for a variety of reasons. Eating disorders are generally secretive and solitary in nature which precludes using information from friends or family to corroborate the self-report. Eating disorders are associated with especially high levels of shame and embarrassment which might also color self-report. Since many of the symptoms and behaviors of eating disorders (especially binge eating and purging) occur frequently while emotionally distressed (Grilo & Shiffman, 1994), it may be difficult for patients to provide accurate retrospective accounts of their behaviors. Fourth, even with high motivation or willingness to report accurately, a number of factors can produce biases including time, memory recall factors, intervening events, and mood states. Laboratory studies allow for careful ongoing observations of these complex phenomena. An obvious potential limitation of laboratory studies concerns their somewhat artificial nature and the uncertain impact of being watched and observed so carefully. This might suggest that participants would presumably decrease the likelihood of "eating naturally" or "binge eating as usual" in such settings. Of course, it is also possible that the demand characteristics and food availability in the laboratory settings could contribute to exaggerating the overeating. Laboratory studies have been revealing in several notable ways.

Laboratory studies have generally found that patients with bulimia nervosa consume impressive amounts of food that are substantially greater than the estimates from studies based on eating naturalistically. Carefully conducted laboratory studies with bulimic inpatients have generally reported average intakes during binge episodes between 3031 kcal (Walsh, Kissileff, Cassidy, & Dantzic, 1989) and 4477 kcal (Kissileff, Walsh, Kral, & Cassidy, 1986). Thus, the average size of binge episodes in laboratory studies is greater than the estimates derived from self-reports of binge eating in naturalistic settings. Laboratory studies have also observed considerable vari-ability both *within* and *between* patients with bulimia nervosa in their binge eating behaviors and associated emotional experiences. Kaye, Gwirtsman, George, Weiss, and Jimerson (1986) studied binge and purge behaviors in 12 women with bulimia on the day after they were admitted to a hospital. In a laboratory setting, the 12 women were provided food and a bathroom and were instructed to binge and purge as they would normally do. Several of the patients had several binge–vomit cycles within the time period of observation. What was clear was the variability between individuals as well as within individuals across multiple binge–vomit cycles in terms of time spent eating, amount and types of food, amount purged, and emotional states before and after the binge–purge cycles.

Two decades of research later, the consensus is that a subjective sense of lack of control is the hallmark criterion for signifying binge eating, but there continues to be less agreement regarding the importance of size or amount of food (Keel, Mayer, & Harnden-Fischer, 2001; Pratt, Niego, & Agras, 1998).

Recurrent inappropriate weight compensatory behaviors

The second criterion for bulimia nervosa is the regular use of extreme or inappropriate compensatory methods to prevent weight gain. This includes behaviors such as self-induced vomiting; misuse of laxatives, diuretics, enemas, or diet pills; severe dieting such as fasting; or excessive vigorous exercise. The DSM-IV also requires (third criterion for bulimia nervosa) that the inappropriate weight compensatory behaviors occur at least twice weekly over the past three months.

Considerable variability exists in the types and frequency of extreme weight compensatory behaviors reported within and across studies. Many patients with bulimia nervosa use more than one method to try to compensate for binge eating and to control their weight. The most common weight compensatory behavior is self-induced vomiting after an episode of binge eating followed by misuse of laxatives. Approximately 80% of patients with bulimia nervosa who seek treatment report self-induced vomiting and roughly 30% report misusing laxatives as their methods of purging calories. Less frequently observed, but not uncommon, is the episodic misuse of diet pills and rarely used are enemas.

After the seminal paper by Russell (1979), studies with community and clinical samples began to examine purging practices. Early studies reported that self-induced vomiting was employed daily by roughly 50% of patients with bulimia (Fairburn & Cooper, 1982; Johnson et al., 1982). Repeated or multiple episodes of self-induced vomiting are not uncommon and can be readily observed even in laboratory settings

(Kaye et al., 1986). Self-induced vomiting, which follows the onset of binge eating on average by one year, is achieved by various means. By far the most common method is the use of fingers to trigger the gag reflex. Many patients are soon able to readily induce vomiting and can do it practically at will without effort. Some patients drink water to facilitate the vomiting. Purging seems to temporarily reduce physical distress from the binge eating and emotional distress including the fear of weight gain, although this relief is eventually replaced by disgust and shame. Nonetheless, in some patients, vomiting appears to become a goal, and these patients will repeatedly vomit or will vomit after eating very small amounts of food. Patients with bulimia nervosa who participated in the treatment study by Agras and colleagues (2000a) reported having substantially more vomiting episodes than binge eating episodes (39 versus 25) in the month prior to beginning treatment. Although rare, some patients take ipecac (a chemical sometimes kept in the medicine cabinet to induce vomiting in case of poisoning), a dangerous practice, to induce vomiting. There is some research indicating greater psychopathology among patients who use multiple methods, particularly laxatives (Hall, Blakey, & Hall, 1992; Pryor, Wiederman, & McGilley, 1996).

The two common nonpurging weight compensatory behaviors include severe dieting or fasting and excessive exercise. These behaviors are a bit more difficult to quantify than the purging behaviors. Patients with bulimia nervosa tend to alternate between periods of severe dietary restriction and periods of binge eating (or binge eating and purging). The restrictive dieting is nearly universal (Johnson et al., 1982; Pyle et al., 1981) and this physiological and psychological deprivation is believed to make patients vulnerable to binge eating (Fairburn, Marcus, & Wilson, 1993b; Grilo & Shiffman, 1994). Although it is unclear how restrictive the dieting needs to be, some researchers have set a strict standard of eight hours of fasting (Fairburn & Cooper, 1993). Excessive exercise is also commonly used by patients with bulimia nervosa. Although studies suggest that extreme exercise in this patient group is less common than seen in anorexia nervosa (Brewerton, Stellefson, Hibbs, Hodges, & Cochrane, 1995b; Davis et al., 1997), roughly one-forth of patients with bulimia nervosa regularly engage in excessive exercise (Brewerton et al., 1995b).

Overevaluation of weight or shape

The fourth criterion, and arguably the core feature, is that weight and shape concerns unduly influence self-evaluation and self-worth. This criterion for BN is more focused than the broader range of body-related disturbances that meet the parallel requirement for AN. Persons with bulimia nervosa place excessive focus and emphasis on body shape and weight for determining their self-worth and self-esteem. Thus, in contrast to the way in which many individuals judge self-worth by considering various important aspects of their lives, persons with bulimia nervosa will rank shape and weight as the highest or amongst the highest factors in determining how they judge themselves.

Subtypes of bulimia nervosa

The DSM-IV (1994) specifies two subtypes of bulimia nervosa, "purging type" and "nonpurging type." The "purging type" regularly engages in self-induced vomiting or the misuse of laxatives, diuretics, or enemas, whereas, the "nonpurging type" uses the other forms of inappropriate weight compensatory behaviors, most notably highly restrictive dieting and excessive exercise. In the later case, the weight is insufficiently low and weight compensatory behaviors insufficient to result in anorexia nervosa. This subtyping scheme has generally received empirical support (Hay, Fairburn, & Doll, 1996) but this is not unequivocal (Sloan, Mizes, & Epstein, 2005; Tobin, Griffing, & Griffing, 1997). Moreover, different subtyping schemes not based on purging have been suggested (Stice & Agras, 1999) and these have received some support (Grilo, 2004; Grilo, Masheb, & Berman, 2001). Different approaches to classifying these eating problems are currently the focus of ongoing debate (Williamson et al., 2005).

Eating disorder not otherwise specified (EDNOS)

Table 1.3 lists the DSM-IV (APA, 1994) diagnostic criteria for eating disorder not otherwise specified (EDNOS). The DSM-IV notes that this category "is for disorders of eating that do not meet the criteria for any specific eating disorder" (APA, 1994; p. 550) and the six examples listed in Table 1.3. Thus, the DSM-IV primarily defines EDNOS in relation to anorexia nervosa and bulimia nervosa by broadening the boundaries (i.e., dropping some criteria). The ICD-10 description of this residual category, labeled "atypical eating disorders" lists six

TABLE 1.3

Eating disorder not otherwise specified (EDNOS): Examples of disorders that do not meet criteria for the specific eating disorder diagnoses (anorexia nervosa or bulimia nervosa)

1. In females, all criteria for anorexia nervosa are met except amenorrhea.
2. All criteria for anorexia nervosa are met except that, despite considerable weight loss, the person's weight is still within "normal" range.
3. All criteria for bulimia nervosa are met except for the frequency (twice weekly) or duration (three months) requirements.
4. Regular inappropriate weight compensatory behaviors by normal weight person after eating small amounts of food (i.e., not binge episodes).
5. Recurrent episodes of chewing and spitting, but not swallowing, large amounts of food.
6. Binge eating disorder, defined as recurrent binge eating without the inappropriate weight compensatory behaviors that define bulimia nervosa.

Six examples included in the *Diagnostic and statistical manual of mental disorders* (4th ed.; *DSM-IV*) published by the American Psychiatric Association (1994). The final example, binge eating disorder, is described more fully as a "research category" and is therefore summarized in Table 1.4.

different categories ("codes"). Like the DSM-IV, two specific types are "atypical anorexia nervosa" and "atypical bulimia nervosa" which are basically broader categories with lessened criteria. For example, the "atypical anorexia nervosa" category in the ICD-10 pretty much resembles the first two examples of EDNOS provided in the DSM-IV (see Table 1.3). A person who presents with a fairly typical constellation of features but is missing a key criterion such as the specific weight loss requirement or the amenorrhea would be given this diagnosis.

The ICD-10 provides a few other codes for atypical eating disorders that are noted here to provide a broader view of this poorly understood residual category that potentially reflects a broad range of disordered eating. A third category included is "overeating associated with other psychological disturbances." This diagnosis can be given in cases where clear psychological motivations exist for the overeating or when distressing events have triggered overeating which has contributed to obesity. It is worth noting here that such psychological views of overeating were common in the American literature for decades (e.g., Richardson, 1946) and were the focus of psychotherapies for obesity (e.g., Stunkard, 1959), but have generally fallen out of favor as potential explanations for obesity in general. This is not to say that such mechanisms or reactions may not exist for certain individuals. A fourth category included is "vomiting associated with other psychological disturbances" and this is distinguished as a separate symptom or phenomenon from the self-induced vomiting as a weight compensatory behavior in bulimia nervosa. The ICD-10 includes little information about two final potential examples, coded as "other eating disorders" and "eating disorders, unspecified."

As will be presented in chapter 4, the residual or other categories in both classification systems (EDNOS and atypical ED) are probably more common than the two formal eating disorders. Unfortunately, they are poorly understood and under-researched. Research efforts following the DSM-IV criteria likely exclude many persons with clinically-meaningful problems but who fail to meet the full criteria for the formal eating disorder diagnoses of AN and BN. Although the DSM-IV also indicates the need for research to consider varied criteria, researchers have been wary to do so for pragmatic reasons (i.e., concerns about getting their studies funded or and eventually published). There is increasing call (e.g., Grilo, Levy, Becker, Edell, & McGlashan, 1996; Fairburn & Bohn, in press; Fairburn & Walsh, 2002) to extend research to a fuller range of patients with clinically-meaningful eating problems. Further research on atypical eating disorders and how to classify them is essential (Mizes & Sloan, 1998).

Binge eating disorder (BED)

Table 1.4 lists the DSM-IV (APA, 1994) criteria for binge eating disorder (BED). Although BED is presently officially considered an example of EDNOS (Table 1.3), BED is also included as a research diagnosis in Appendix B of the DSM-IV, which lists "criteria sets and axes provided for further study (p. 703)." This research category was included in the DSM-IV given findings from two large multi-site field trials (Spitzer et al., 1992, 1993) and various other research efforts (Yanovski, 1993) suggesting the potential utility and distinctiveness of this diagnosis. Although this addition was not without controversy (Fairburn, Welch, & Hay, 1993c; Fichter, Quadflieg, & Brandl, 1993), it seemed to foster research attention on what now appears to be a significant clinical problem (Wilfley, Wilson, & Agras, 2003).

The research diagnosis of BED requires recurrent episodes of binge eating. It is important to begin by noting that the fifth criterion is that the person does not regularly use inappropriate weight compensatory behaviors and does not meet current criteria for anorexia nervosa or bulimia nervosa. A description of the core features follows.

TABLE 1.4

Binge eating disorder: Definition and diagnostic criteria

A.   Recurrent binge eating.
B.   The binge eating episodes are associated with at least three of the following five behaviors: very rapid eating, eating until uncomfortably full, eating large quantities in the absence of hunger, eating alone because of embarrassment due to the amount of eating, and feeling disgust, depressed, or guilty after the overeating.
C.   Marked distress about the binge eating.
D.   Binge eating occurs at least two days per week for six months.
E.   No regular use of inappropriate weight compensatory behaviors and does not meet criteria for anorexia nervosa or bulimia nervosa.

Based on the five criteria and subtyping in the *Diagnostic and statistical manual of mental disorders* (4th ed.; *DSM-IV*) published by the American Psychiatric Association (1994).

Recurrent binge eating

Binge eating is defined – as in bulimia nervosa – as eating unusually large quantities of food in a discrete period of time while experiencing a clear sense of lack of control. The second criterion requires that at least three of five behavioral indicators are associated with the binge eating. These behavioral indicators of impaired control over eating include: very rapid eating, eating until uncomfortably full, eating large quantities of food despite not being hungry, eating alone because of embarrassment due to the amount of eating, and feeling disgust, depressed, or guilty after the eating. The research diagnosis also requires that the binge eating occurs at least twice weekly over the past six months. The research criteria and description of binge eating are noteworthy in several respects when compared with those for BN. A brief review of issues and research on different aspects of binge eating in this patient group follows.

First, the requirement for BED that binge episodes occur two days per week is different from the requirement of two episodes per week for BN. In patients with BN, the binge eating frequently follows a clear period of food restriction and is usually terminated by either purging or by the re-establishment of strict dietary restriction. In contrast, the eating habits of persons with BED are much more amorphous than those with BN. Many patients with BED report days with ongoing eating (sometimes referred to as "grazing") during which the overeating "shifts" into binge eating and total loss of control. Thus, it is sometimes difficult to determine whether separate or discrete binge episodes occurred on certain days. Because of these observations, the research and diagnostic practice became to determine the number of days on which binge episodes occurred. The frequency stipulation of twice weekly was adopted to parallel to BN criterion. The intent here was to identify a clinically-meaningful patient group by preventing the diagnosis from being given to persons who infrequently binge eat (Wilson, 1992).

The DSM-IV acknowledged the clear need for research to address these methods to determine the criterion of recurrent binge eating. First, laboratory studies have demonstrated that patients with BED exhibit objectively non-normative eating behaviors (Walsh & Boudreau, 2003). In such laboratory settings, discrete binge episodes are observable and obese patients with BED ate significantly more than obese comparison patients during meals and when instructed to binge (Guss, Kissileff, Devlin, Zimmerli, & Walsh, 2002; Yanovski et al., 1992). In these laboratory studies with BED patients, average intakes during binge episodes have averaged roughly 3000 kcal (Yanovski et al., 1992). Naturalistic studies have also found that although patients with BED and BN eat similar quantities of food during binge episodes (Fitzgibbon & Blackman, 2000; Mitchell et al., 1999), there exist differences in the quality or nature of the binge eating. Patients with BN consume a greater proportion of carbo-hydrates than patients with BED (Fitzgibbon & Blackman, 2000) while patients with BED report enjoying the food more and experi-encing less distress than the BN patients as a consequence of the binge eating (Mitchell et al., 1999). Collectively, these findings support aspects of the validity of this eating disorder category.

Second, studies have found that patients with BED can provide reports of binge eating episodes about as reliably as days during which they had binge eating episodes (Grilo, Masheb, Lozano-Blanco, & Barry, 2004a; Grilo, Masheb, & Wilson, 2001a, 2001b; Reas, Grilo, & Masheb, 2006). These findings suggest the feasibility of trying to assess the frequency of binge eating episodes, rather than relying on just counting days with binges. Clinically, this seems logical and advantageous. Since the typical binge episode tends to be quite large in quantity, it seems important to keep track of how many times they happen. This logic is further supported by research demonstrating that in patients with BED, larger binge episodes are positively cor-related with greater obesity. Also, there is no a priori reason to view a persistent weekly pattern of two days each with one binge episode as signifying a greater problem than a persistent weekly pattern of one day with two binge episodes.

Third, as in the case for BN, the twice-weekly criterion for BED is arbitrary. It was selected to prevent the diagnoses from being given to persons who infrequently binge. Research to date with BED across community and clinical settings has suggested, much like the case for BN, variability in the frequency of binge eating between and within individuals over time. Recent clinical studies have reported that patients with BED who seek treatment report roughly five binges per week (Grilo et al., 2001a, 2001b). These average frequencies do not appear very different from those observed in community studies of BED using similar assessment methods (Grilo, Lozano, & Masheb, 2005; Pike, Dohm, Striegel-Moore, Wilfley, & Fairburn, 2001), although there is some suggestion that those who seek treatment have greater severity (Wilfley, Pike, Dohm, Striegel-Moore, & Fairburn, 2001). Several studies that examined the utility of the twice-weekly requirement in BED found no important differences in the clinical features of persons who binge at least once weekly versus twice or more weekly (Elder, Grilo, Masheb, Rothschild, Burke-Martindale, & Brody, 2006; Striegel-Moore, Wilson, Wilfley, Elder, & Brownell, 1998; Striegel-Moore, Dohm, Solomon, Fairburn, Pike, & Wilfley, 2000a).

Fourth, the duration or time frame of six months of recurrent binge eating as associated distress is a departure from the three-month duration criterion for BN (i.e., for regular binge eating and weight compensatory behaviors) and AN (i.e., for amenorrhea). This arbitrary criterion was based on some concerns regarding the instability or potentially transient nature of the features of BED. Using data from a national sample of over 3000 adult women in the United States, Dansky and colleagues (1998) reported that using a three-month requirement would have resulted in a 1.6% prevalence estimate versus the 1.0% prevalence estimate using the six-month requirement. The value of this criterion remains uncertain.

Marked distress

The third criterion requires that the binge eating is associated with marked distress. This criterion is frequently evidenced by patients' reports of unpleasant physical and emotional feelings during and after the binge eating. Although the binge eating may initially reduce negative feelings, such effects are transient and are rapidly replaced by uncomfortable feelings of physical fullness and intense disgust and guilt. Many patients cite the loss of control itself as terribly upsetting and others have strong concerns regarding the recurrent binge eating on their body weight and shape.

This criterion seems to simply reflect the universal requirement by the DSM-IV for psychiatric diagnoses to have negative impact. In sharp contrast to the formal eating disorder diagnoses of AN and BN, there is no specific attitudinal or cognitive criterion for BED involving overevaluation of centrality of weight or shape concerns. A significant body of research has documented that obese patients with BED have significantly greater dysfunctional attitudes and overevaluation of weight/shape than their non-binge-eating obese peers (Allison, Grilo, Masheb, & Stunkard, 2005; Grilo, 1998). Obese BED patients have greater shape and weight concerns than obese patients with other forms of disordered eating such as night eating syndrome (Allison et al., 2005) and have levels similar in intensity to those of patients with BN (Masheb & Grilo, 2000; Barry, Grilo, & Masheb, 2003; Wilfley, Schwartz, Spurrell, & Fairburn, 2000). Importantly, the intensity of dysfunctional attitudes regarding eating, shape, and weight do not differ between BED patients who are obese versus not obese (Masheb & Grilo, 2000).

Obesity

Obesity is a physical problem and is classified as a general medical condition in the ICD-10. Since it has not been consistently associated with either a behavioral or a psychological problem, it is not included in the DSM-IV. Obesity is defined as excess adipose (fat) tissue that results from excess energy intake relative to energy expenditure. Overweight refers to excess body weight above some standard ("ideal") for height. Excess weight does not always reflect excess fat. For example, some muscular athletes may be overweight but not necessarily obese.

"Ideal" weights

The first approach widely used to define "healthy" body weights came from the Metropolitan Life Insurance Company, which published the famous 1959 tables listing "ideal" weights. These tables, which were widely used for years, listed "ideal" weights separately for men and women aged 25 to 59 years divided into small, medium, and large body frames. These ideal weights were defined using the lowest mortality rates based on data from roughly 5 million insurance policies obtained from 26 insurance companies in the United States and Canada between 1935 and 1953. These tables, although impressive in their scope and predictive utility, were limited in several ways. Since they were based on persons with life insurance policies, they were limited to primarily wealthier, healthier, better educated, and mostly white persons living in these two countries. These tables also excluded cases of certain major diseases (cardiovascular disease, diabetes, and certain cancers) and did not provide information on smoking. Collectively, these factors probably biased the tables towards listing higher ideal weights.

In 1983, the Metropolitan Life Insurance Company published a second set of weight for height tables based on data from over 4 million insurance policies issued between 1950 and 1975. Of note, the weights listed for ideal (with the lowest mortality) in the 1983 tables were higher than those in the 1959 tables. This is generally attributed to the potential bias introduced by smoking status, since the negative health consequences are not experienced until years later.

Body mass index (BMI)

The second major, and current, approach involves the use of body mass index (BMI) instead of ideal or relative weights. BMI is defined as weight (in kilograms) divided by height (in meters squared). Table 1.5 shows the method for calculating BMI and includes the English formula. Although the BMI is not perfect, it is easy to determine and correlates roughly .9 with direct measurements of body fat. It is important to note that the BMI may overestimate obesity in muscular or athletic persons and may underestimate obesity in older persons who have lost lean tissue with age and decreased exercise.

For years, overweight was defined as having a BMI $\geq$ 27 and obesity was defined as having a BMI $\geq$ 30. The National Heart, Lung and Blood Institute, together with the National Institute of Diabetes and Digestive and Kidney Diseases, issued the first set of federal guidelines for addressing obesity in 1998. These federal guidelines were critically reviewed by 115 health experts and were endorsed by representatives from 54 organizations with interest and involvement in relevant issues. The NHLBI (1998) *Clinical guidelines on the identification, evaluation, and treatment of overweight and obesity* adopted a lower threshold for overweight (i.e., BMI $\geq$ 25) and retained the BMI $\geq$ 30 as signifying obesity. Table 1.5 lists the entire classification system based on BMI, ranging from "underweight" (below 18.5) through "extreme obesity" (above 40.0). These guidelines have also been adopted by the World Health Organization. The uniform

TABLE 1.5
Obesity: Body mass index – calculation and classification of weight and obesity

Body mass index (BMI)	Classification
< 18.5	Underweight
18.5–24.9	Normal weight
25.0–29.9	Overweight
30.0–34.9	Obesity (Class I)
35.0–39.9	Obesity (Class II)
> 40.0	Extreme obesity (Class III)

Body mass index (BMI) calculation
BMI is defined (kg/m^2)
BMI is calculated as weight (kilograms) divided by height (meters squared)
BMI English formula = [weight (pounds) divided by height (inches squared)] times 703

Classification of weight and obesity levels by body mass index based on the National Heart, Lung, and Blood Institute (NHLBI, 1998) guidelines.

method of classification is facilitating research and comparison of findings internationally.

The change in the definition of overweight in 1998 (lowering of BMI from 27 to 25) reflected important research findings. Data from several landmark longitudinal studies, including the American Cancer Society Cohort Study, the Harvard Alumni Study, the Health Professionals Follow-up Study, and the Nurse's Health Study, consistently support the establishment of "healthy" weight at the BMI levels between 18.5 and 25.0. An impressive body of evidence suggests that overweight (defined as BMI $\geq$ 25) is associated with increased risk for morbidity and mortality from multiple causes (to be described in chapter 6). Also, the continuing increases in the prevalence of obesity throughout the world suggested the need to identify potential weight problems at an earlier stage.

Upper-body obesity

In addition to BMI, it is particularly important to consider the distribution of fat. Abdominal fat distribution (upper-body or android-type) is associated with substantially greater morbidity and mortality than lower-body (gynoid-type) obesity. Men are more likely than women to have abdominal fat distribution, but it is associated with increased medical problems regardless of gender (Folsom et al., 2000; Stamler, Wentworth, & Neaton, 1986). Thus, although a BMI $\geq$ 30 is associated with sharp increase in health risks, waist circumference is a strong independent predictor of health risk, especially cardiovascular disease (Rexrode et al., 1998). Waist circumference provides an adequate estimate of intra-abdominal obesity, which would otherwise require sophisticated and expensive testing (Lichtenbelt & Fogelholm, 1992). In chapter 6, assessment and consideration of medical risk by both obesity level (BMI) and type (i.e., abdominal obesity) will be discussed.

Disordered eating versus eating disorders

As noted above, in the psychiatric classification systems, eating disorders refer to clinically-meaningful behavioral or psychological patterns having to do with eating or weight that are associated with distress, disability, or with substantially increased risk of morbidity or mortality. Fairburn and Walsh (2002) suggested a more specific definition of an eating disorder as "a persistent disturbance of eating behavior or behavior intended to control weight, which significantly impairs physical health or psychosocial functioning" (p. 171). These general definitions raise a few logical questions. First, what about disturbed eating or "non-normative" eating without associated distress or impairment (Tanofsky-Kraff & Yanovski, 2004)? Second, what about overeating in persons who are obese and are either at risk for obesity-related complications (e.g., pre-diabetic) or already have obesity-related complications that can be reversed by modest weight loss (hypertension, some cases of type II diabetes)?

Tanofsky-Kraff and Yanovski (2004) recently argued for the distinction between "eating disorders" and disordered eating, which they termed "non-normative" eating patterns without associated distress or impairment. They argued that although non-normative eating patterns may not warrant a psychiatric diagnosis, they may be quite important because of how they influence body weight and health. Greater clinical and research attention paid to different forms of disordered eating may ultimately improve our understanding of both eating disorders and obesity.

Interestingly, from a historical perspective, some of these views are not entirely new but seem to have surfaced again. Early clinical views of obesity emphasized psychological problems. Obesity was thought to reflect some form of an underlying psychological problem (Richardson, 1946). These views were eventually replaced, at least partly, by the belief that obesity reflected disordered eating.

Stunkard's astute clinical observations of two forms of disordered eating in obese persons, night eating (Stunkard, Grace, & Wolf, 1955) and binge eating (Stunkard, 1959) did not stimulate much research attention until many years later. The prevailing perspective that evolved was that people became obese simply by eating too much (Ferster, Nurnberger, & Levitt, 1962) and this led to the application of learning and behavioral principles to combat overeating (Stuart, 1967). This perhaps simplistic view was eventually replaced by multimodal perspectives of obesity comprising complex combinations of genetic, biological, psychological, behavioral, and societal influences. Interestingly, recent years have witnessed resurgence in attention paid to the role of disordered eating (particularly binge eating and night eating) in some cases of obesity. With this context in mind, a specific type of non-normative eating problem – termed night eating syndrome – will be described here.

Night eating syndrome

Night eating syndrome (NES), first described by Stunkard and his colleagues (1955), was initially defined as morning anorexia, evening hyperphagia (overeating), and sleep disturbance that was exacerbated during periods of stress. NES was distinguished, in part, from several "nocturnal sleep-related eating disorders" (Schenck & Mahowald, 1994). In contrast to the sleep-disorders, patients with NES are awake and fully aware of their eating activities at night. The definition of NES continues to evolve with emerging research findings (de Zwaan, Burgard, Schenck, & Mitchell, 2003; Grilo & Masheb, 2004; O'Reardon et al., 2004) but is not included in the DSM-IV. Since the initial descriptions, the requirement of awakenings with nocturnal ingestions has been added (Birketvedt et al., 1999), but different researchers have used varying definitions for "night-time" (e.g., 6pm, 8pm, or "after the evening meal") and for "amount of food intake." Recent analyses by Allison, Grilo, Masheb, & Stunkard (2005) suggest the specific predictive utility of two features: (1) eating 25% or more of the daily total caloric intake after the evening meal; (2) having awakenings with nocturnal eating at least half of the days.

Summary

Diverse patterns of abnormal eating behaviors and beliefs about eating and body shape and disordered eating exist across the entire continuum of weight (from underweight to obese). It is often difficult to determine what is "non-normative" and how, or where, to draw a line between a concern, a problem, and a disorder. Eating disorders are clinical entities (classified as psychiatric disorders) that negatively impact on quality of life. AN, the least common but most serious problem, refers to a dangerously underweight condition fueled by severe body image disturbances and sustained by severe dieting and weight control methods. BN, a relatively uncommon problem most often found in average weight persons, is characterized by frequent fluctuations between dietary restraint or control, binge eating, and inappropriate weight control methods such as purging. Obesity is a physical or a medical problem and is defined by excess fat. Obesity is a serious health problem (not simply an aesthetic issue) that, unlike AN and BN, is quite common and increasingly in prevalence, and is one of the leading causes of morbidity and mortality. A variety of disordered eating problems exist (such as binge eating and night eating) that cut across all weight categories.

The epidemiology and nature of eating and weight disorders 2

Epidemiology and distribution of eating disorders

Figure 2.1 is a representation of the relationships of eating disorders and eating, weight, and body image concerns. The schematic representation is intended to convey certain diagnostic relationships and serve as a useful heuristic about the relative prevalence of eating disorders. Eating *disorders* refer to clinically-meaningful behavioral or psychological patterns that are associated with distress or disability or with increased risk of morbidity or mortality. It can sometimes be difficult to determine when a behavior becomes non-normative or a concern becomes distressing and interferes with functioning. As Figure 2.1 shows, whereas eating *disorders* are relatively uncommon, there exists a plethora of eating, weight, and body image concerns that are very common. Figure 2.1 does not include obesity, which is described separately later in this chapter. Obesity is a very prevalent physical problem that is associated in complex and highly variable ways to many of these eating and body image concerns as well as to eating disorders.

Diagnostically, anorexia nervosa (AN) "trumps" bulimia nervosa (BN) which, in turn "trumps" binge eating disorder (BED) and other examples of the eating disorder not otherwise specified (EDNOS) residual category of eating disorders. The diagnostic requirements described in chapter 1 specify exclusion rules to result in these apparently distinct groupings. The dotted lines are intended to reflect some ambiguities in the boundaries because of how some criteria are interpreted. As is noted in several places in this book, studies have found complex patterns of migration ("diagnostic crossover") across these diagnostic groupings over time. Such diagnostic crossover is not included in Figure 2.1. In terms of prevalence, Figure 2.1 shows that AN is the least common eating disorder followed by bulimia nervosa.

Figure 2.1.
Schematic
representation of
eating disorders and
concerns.

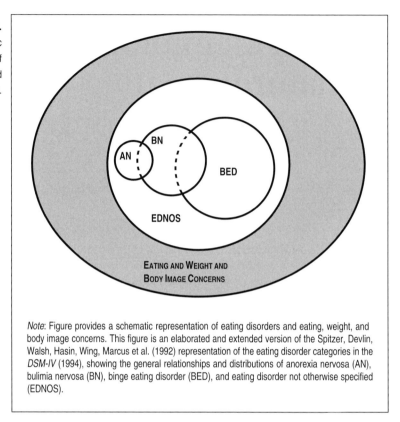

Note: Figure provides a schematic representation of eating disorders and eating, weight, and body image concerns. This figure is an elaborated and extended version of the Spitzer, Devlin, Walsh, Hasin, Wing, Marcus et al. (1992) representation of the eating disorder categories in the *DSM-IV* (1994), showing the general relationships and distributions of anorexia nervosa (AN), bulimia nervosa (BN), binge eating disorder (BED), and eating disorder not otherwise specified (EDNOS).

BED is thought to be considerably more prevalent than both AN and BN. It is generally though that EDNOS is by far the most prevalent eating disorder although this is based on very little research.

Prevalence of eating disorders

There are several measures for describing the frequency of eating disorders. Prevalence refers to the total number of cases in a population. This is generally the most useful measure since it tells you how many people have a disorder and may require services. Incidence refers to the number of new cases (or at least when cases are detected) in a population per year or per some specified time period. Incidence rates are generally estimated from cases presenting to health centers and in the case of eating disorders there have not been any studies of incidence in any population.

Prevalence studies with eating disorders are difficult to perform and the findings must be viewed cautiously for several reasons. Eating disorders, particularly AN and BN, are rare and this results in the need for very large studies to detect cases. Even the largest studies conducted to date have only included approximately 3000 subjects, which may be insufficient to arrive at a solid estimate. This difficulty is further complicated by the secrecy and denial that are characteristic of many patients with eating disorders. Researchers have relied on a variety of methods for gathering data to generate estimates of eating disorders. This includes examination of case registers, "two-stage" screen/interview studies, and special population or high-risk studies. Each of these has limitations. Each of these approaches has advantages and disadvantages and can only be viewed as methods to obtain estimates given the absence of more definitive epidemiological research in this area. The reader is referred to Hoek (1991, 1993, 2002; Hoek & van Hoeken, 2003) for detailed descriptions of these issues and for critical reviews of the literature.

Reviews of the available studies, keeping in mind the limitations noted above, have resulted in fairly consistent estimates of prevalence for the eating disorders (Fairburn & Beglin, 1990; Hoek & van Hoeken, 2003). For AN, the average prevalence estimate across studies (that used a two-stage screening and assessment method) reviewed critically by Hoek & van Hoeken (2003) is 0.3% among young females. Studies conducted in Europe revealed similar estimates of prevalence, generally about 0.3% of young females. Hoek (1993), in an earlier review of prevalence studies of anorexia nervosa conducted using criteria from an earlier edition of the DSM, also reported an average rate of roughly 0.3%. One important population-based study is worth specific mention since is offers an especially systematic approach to determining prevalence. Lucas, Beard, O'Fallon, and Kurland (1991) searched case and medical records of health care providers for diagnoses and symptoms of AN for all persons residing in the community of Rochester, Minnesota. They identified 181 possible cases of AN for the time period between 1935 and 1985. This study was subsequently updated by searching all medical records through 1989 resulting in a total of 208 cases of AN (193 in females and 15 in males).

For BN, the average prevalence rate across two-stage survey studies is 1.0% in young women (Hoek & van Hoeken, 2003). It is noteworthy that two major reviews conducted 13 years apart concluded that the prevalence of bulimia is 1% in young women (Fairburn & Beglin, 1990; Hoek & van Hoeken, 2003). For BED, a specific example of EDNOS, rough estimates place its prevalence between 1% and 3% (Grilo, 2002; Hay, 1998; Johnson, Spitzer, & Williams, 2001; Westenhoefer, 2001). Dansky and colleagues (1998), using data from a national sample of over 3000 women in the United States, reported a 1.0% prevalence estimate.

The prevalence of EDNOS or atypical eating disorders in the community is unknown. Fairburn and Bohn (in press), in their review, concluded that EDNOS is the most common eating disorder diagnosis given in most outpatient clinical settings, except for research clinics that recruit for or attract patients with specific eating disorders for studies. Specifically, Fairburn and Bohn (in press) noted that the average prevalence of EDNOS was 60% (versus 14.5% for anorexia nervosa and 25.5% for bulimia nervosa) in four adult clinical outpatient samples with eating disorders. For example, Turner and Bryant-Waugh (2004) reported that 70.5% of a series of eating disordered patients seen at a community center received the EDNOS diagnosis. The high rates of EDNOS in clinical samples suggest that these forms of eating disorders are also common in the community and likely to be more prevalent than anorexia nervosa and bulimia nervosa, although this awaits research confirmation.

A few studies of the prevalence of specific eating disorders have also reported prevalence estimates for "partial" or "subthreshold" levels of AN and BN. Wittchen, Nelson, and Lachner (1998), for example, reported that an additional 1.5% of females and 0.4% of males would receive a diagnosis of AN and an additional 1.5% of females and 0.6% of males would receive a diagnosis of BN if these two diagnoses required one fewer criterion. Regular binge eating (defined as overeating with a loss of control at least a few times weekly and feeling upset about the overeating) was reported by 3.1% of girls and 0.9% of boys in Project Eat (Eating Among Teens), a population-based study of 4746 adolescents in Minnesota public middle and high schools (Ackard, Neumark-Sztainer, Story, & Perry, 2003).

Prevalence of eating, weight, and body-related concerns

The prevalence of eating, weight, and body-image related concerns is generally thought to be high, but quantification of such concerns is difficult due to the obvious difficulties in defining and measuring these diverse problem areas. In general, the prevalence of unhealthy eating behaviors and weight control behaviors are obviously much higher than the prevalence rates for the various eating disorders noted above. Many of these potentially problematic behaviors have occurred in the vast majority of people from time to time. It is difficult, however, to determine at what point diet and weight loss behaviors no longer reflect healthy efforts but instead reflect problems and become potentially harmful. A different challenge is that self-reports of dieting are often not reflective of actual behaviors. A substantial body of research has found, for example, that while many persons report that they are dieting, their day-to-day behaviors do not reveal behavioral attempts to decrease eating or increase activity (Neumark-Sztainer, Jeffery, & French, 1997). In addition, even relatively subtle differences in the wording used to ask about these various behaviors can influence the results considerably and contribute to variability across studies (Brener, Grunbaum, Kann, McManus, & Ross, 2004).

When increased specifics about the behaviors (e.g., quantity, intensity, frequency, and duration) are considered when determining occurrence, the estimates are decreased. So, while the majority of women may report having experienced "binge eating," the frequency falls considerably when additional requirements (unusually large quantity of food, clear loss of control, regular pattern over a certain amount of time) are considered. A different example concerns night eating. Awakening in the middle of the night to eat ("night eating") is not uncommon and has been reported to occur occasionally in up to one-fourth of certain clinical samples (Grilo & Masheb, 2004). The prevalence of night eating syndrome (which requires a certain amount of night eating) is much less common, however, and has been estimated at roughly 1.5% in the general population (Rand, Macgregor, & Stunkard, 1997). With these general issues and examples as context, a brief overview of what is known about the prevalence of selected eating, weight, and body image concerns follows.

Attempting to lose weight

The prevalence of attempting to lose weight in the US has been studied in several large and ongoing national studies. Serdula, Mokdad, Williamson, Galuska, Mendleinm and Heath (1999), based on data for 107,804 adults obtained by a random telephone survey as part of the Behavioral Risk Factor Surveillance System, estimated the prevalence of attempting to lose weight was 28.8% in men and 43.6% in women. Interestingly, among those who reported that they were attempting to lose weight, a common strategy (34.9% of men and 40% of women) was to eat less fat but not fewer calories. Moreover, only 21.5% of men and 19.4% of women reported that they were also engaging in at least 150 minutes of leisure-time physical activity per week. More recent analyses of the Behavioral Risk Factor Surveillance System study updated in 2000 with over 184,000 US adults revealed very similar prevalence estimates for dieting and general weight control practices (Bish, Blanck, Serdula, Marcus, Kohl, & Khan, 2005). Kruger, Galuska, Serdula, and Jones (2004) reported similar findings based on data from the 1998 National Health Interview Survey, which involved face-to-face interviews of a nationally representative sample of 32,440 adults in the United States. Thus, while many adults report that they are trying to lose weight, even more adults are overweight (see below) and thus should be trying to control their weight, and only a minority of those who say they are trying to lose weight are actually restricting calories and increasing physical activity.

The prevalence of dieting and weight control behaviors is even higher among adolescents than adults. Grunbaum and colleagues (2002, 2004) have reported relevant data obtained for representative samples of high school students throughout the US as part of the Youth Risk Behavior Surveillance System (YRBS). The most recent data from the YRBS (Grunbaum et al., 2004), which is conducted every two years, revealed that overall 13.5% of these adolescents were classified as overweight and 29.6% described themselves as over-weight (36.1% of girls versus 23.5% of boys). Overall, 43.8% reported that they were trying to lose weight; a higher percentage of girls (59.3%) than boys (29.1%) and a higher percentage of white (44.8%) and hispanic (49.4%) than black (34.7%) adolescents. Neumark-Sztainer, Croll, Story, Hannan, French, and Perry (2002a), in the Project EAT Study, reported that roughly 85% of adolescent girls and 70% of adolescent boys reported "healthy" weight control behaviors. Neumark-Sztainer et al. (2002a) found that most overweight teen-agers also perceived themselves as overweight and actually reported using healthy weight control behaviors. Thus, dieting seems nearly universal among adolescents.

Unhealthy behaviors and body image concerns

Project EAT (Neumark-Sztainer et al., 2002a) estimated the prevalence of unhealthy weight control behaviors was to be 57% for adolescent girls and 33% for adolescent boys. These behaviors were reported by a sample of adolescents in which roughly one-third of both girls and boys were either overweight or obese. Fifty-four percent of girls and 74% of boys reported at least moderate levels of body dissatisfaction. In contrast, girls reported higher levels of caring about or concern about trying to control their weight than did boys. Three large-scale surveys published in *Psychology Today* examined body image in 1972, 1985, and 1996 (Berscheid, Walster, & Bohrnstedt, 1973; Cash, Winstead, & Janda, 1986; Garner, 1997). These surveys provided general data suggesting that both men and women are frequently unhappy with various aspects of their bodies although women consistently report substantially greater body dissatisfaction than men. Perhaps the best attempt to quantify the prevalence of body image dissatisfaction comes from a longstanding program of body image research performed by Cash, Morrow, Hrabosky, and Perry (2004). Cash et al. (2004), based on scores on an established and normed multidimensional measure of body image, estimated that body dissatisfaction is experienced by 29% of white women, 17% of black women, and 16% of white men.

Consistent with those strong concerns about weight and body dissatisfaction, extreme weight control practices (defined as vomiting or taking diet pills, laxatives, or diuretics during the past year) were reported by 12.4% of adolescent girls and by 4.6% of adolescent boys. The prevalence of having vomited to lose weight during the past year was 6.8% for adolescent girls and 2.4% for adolescent boys. The prevalence of these extreme weight control behaviors was highest among overweight teenagers. Indeed, extreme weight control behaviors were reported by 18% of obese girls and 6% of obese boys. The most recent data from the YRBS (Grunbaum et al., 2004) revealed generally similar findings regarding the prevalence of problematic weight control behaviors. The YRBS found that 13.3% of adolescents reported having fasted (gone without eating for at least 24 hours), 9.2% reported taking diet pills without a physician's advice, and 6.0% had vomited or taken laxatives during the previous month in order to lose weight.

Are eating disorders increasing in prevalence?

Epidemiologic research does not suggest much of an increase in the prevalence of anorexia nervosa. What has clearly increased is the

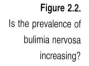

Figure 2.2.
Is the prevalence of
bulimia nervosa
increasing?

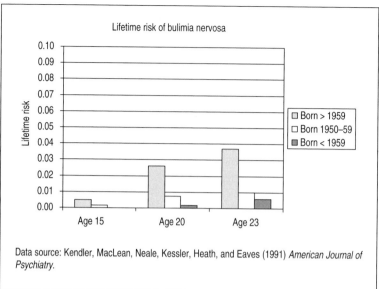

Data source: Kendler, MacLean, Neale, Kessler, Heath, and Eaves (1991) *American Journal of Psychiatry.*

registered incidence (i.e., new cases presenting for treatment) since 1935 (Lucas, Crowson, O'Fallon, & Melton, 1999). Hoek and van Hoeken (2003), in an analysis using combined data from several European countries, concluded that the incidence of AN increased substantially until the 1970s, after which it appears to have stabilized. This increase in identified cases probably reflects greater awareness and identification of the problem by health care professionals. The prevalence and incidence of AN are believed to have remained relatively constant during the past few decades.

In contrast to AN, there is more evidence suggesting that the prevalence of BN has increased over the past few decades. For example, Figure 2.2 shows data from a study by Kendler and colleagues (1991) suggesting that persons born after 1960 have a slightly higher rate of developing BN than those born before 1960. There are some reports that BN is becoming more prevalent in non-Caucasian groups (Crago, Shisslak, & Estes, 1996; Warheit, Langer, Zimmerman, & Biafora, 1993). Although there are fewer studies of the incidence of BN, three studies that used population-based reviews of medical records in three different countries reported very similar findings suggesting an annual incidence rate of approximately 12 per 100,000 (Hoek et al., 1995; Soundy, Lucas, Suman, & Melton, 1995; Turnbull, Ward, Treasure, Jick, & Derby, 1996). Incidence rates for

BN rose sharply soon after the diagnosis was included in the classification system in 1980 and were estimated to be approximately 30 to 50 per 100,000 (Soundy et al., 1995; Turnbull et al., 1996) for 10- to 40-year-old females. Thus, for BN there is some evidence of increasing prevalence and clear evidence of increasing incidence. The increasing incidence may reflect changes in the diagnostic system, greater awareness and better methods for detecting problems, and wider availability of resources and treatments. It is generally thought, however, that the registered incidence is an underestimate of the true rate given the secrecy and ease of hiding the problem.

Are eating, dieting, and body image problems increasing in prevalence?

Problematic eating and dieting behaviors do not appear to be increasing in prevalence, and the best available research suggests that they may be abating slightly over the past 20 years. A brief overview of findings from three important methodologically sound studies using complementary sampling methods follows.

Heatherton, Nichols, Mahamedi, and Keel (1995) examined the eating and dieting behaviors and problems of 625 women and 276 men attending a specific college in 1982. Ten years later, a nearly identical survey was administered to 564 women and 235 men attending the same college. Significant reductions in the frequencies of problematic eating, binge eating, vomiting, diuretic use, diet pill use, and disordered attitudes about shape and weight were observed from 1982 to 1992. Inspection of the YRBS data during the period of time between 1991 and 2003 (Grunbaum et al., 2004) does not reveal recent significant short-term trends or changes in the various eating and problematic weight control practices. During this time period, however, there does appear to be an increase in the rates of physical inactivity and unbalanced nutrition (eating too few fruits and veg- etables). Westenhoefer (2001) found that the prevalence of bulimic behaviors and extreme weight control practices declined slightly from 1990 to 1997 in Germany. Westenhoefer (2001) compared the prevalence of these behaviors in a representative sample of 4285 Germans assessed in 1997 to those reported by a representative survey with 1773 Germans assessed in 1990 with the same measures. The rate of severe binge eating twice weekly dropped from 3.1% to 2.4% in men and from 2.3% to 1.3% in women. Extreme weight control behaviors, such as self-induced vomiting, use of laxatives, appetite suppressants and diuretics, dieting, and exercise remained about the same or dropped slightly.

What about body image? It is widely believed that negative body image has increased over time commensurate with the pervasive bombardment of idealized body shapes across different media coupled with the increases in average body weight and obesity. The three *Psychology Today* surveys are frequently cited as support for increasing body image concerns in our culture. Feingold and Mazzella (1998) reviewed 222 studies on gender differences in body image conducted over a 50-year period. These researchers noted that reports of body dissatisfaction between men and women became increasingly disparate (higher in women) over time. Feingold and Mazzella's (1998) conclusion was that either women's body images worsened over time (but not so for men) or that women's body images worsened more quickly than men. Two strong studies have since been performed with impressive evidence suggesting that overall body image dissatisfaction has stabilized or improved slightly during the past 20 years. Heatherton and colleagues (1995) reported lower body image concerns, despite heavier weights, in their sample of 1992 college students than for their sample of 1982 students. Cash et al. (2004), using sophisticated assessments of body image, examined changes in multiple aspects of body image among 3127 college students cross-sectionally from 1983 to 2001. The prevalence of body dissatisfaction among white women increased until the early 1990s. After the early 1990s, the prevalence of body dissatisfaction decreased among both white and black women, despite higher average body weights. Body image among men appeared stable during this 19-year period. Collectively, these findings suggest that although body image concerns are not uncommon, the prevalence of dissatisfaction may actually be decreasing among women and remaining stable among men despite continued increases in body weight.

Distribution of eating disorders

Eating disorders are not distributed randomly in the population. In fact, eating disorders have rather extreme distributions. Young females are by far the most vulnerable group. Only 5% to 10% of patients with eating disorders in clinical settings are male, and the gender discrepancy is even greater for the specific AN and BN diagnoses. This gender discrepancy is one of the most extreme of any medical or psychiatric problem (Andersen & Holman, 1997). The nature of the age distribution is also notable. AN is distributed most frequently in adolescents although it is also found in young adults. BN is distributed most frequently in young adults although it is also found in adolescents. Although there are increasing reports of both AN and BN in middle adulthood and later, these eating disorders are still far more common in younger people. Both AN and BN are predominantly found in westernized and industrialized countries and are primarily seen in Caucasian groups. Even within the US, AN and BN are much less common in ethnic minority groups. In terms of social class, AN appears to be more common in higher socioeconomic status (SES) groups while BN appears to be evenly distributed across SES groups. Collectively, these overall findings about the extreme distribution of AN and BN by gender, ethnicity, and culture have resulted in frequent description of these eating disorders as "culture-bound syndromes." See Text Box 2.1 for a study of anorexia nervosa in Curacao demonstrating the role of sociocultural factors.

The distribution of BED appears very different than that of AN and BN (Grilo, 2002). Unlike those eating disorders, BED is not uncommon in men, with studies generally suggesting a 3:1 ratio of women to men (Spitzer et al., 1992), nor is it uncommon in minority groups (see Grilo, Lozano, & Masheb, 2005; Pike et al., 2001; Striegel-Moore et al., 2000b; Yanovski, 1993). BED seems to have an older age of onset and is associated with a much older age at presentation for treatment. Most treatment studies for BED find most patients to be between 30 and 50 years of age and report an average age of roughly 43 years (Grilo et al., 2005b). Even naturalistic studies with community-based samples suggest that BED is associated with an older age than is typical for bulimia nervosa (Fairburn, Cooper, Doll, Norman, & O'Connor, 2000).

Distribution of eating, dieting, and body image problems

Eating, dieting, and body image problems are not distributed randomly in the population although these concerns are found with fewer of the disparities seen for the eating disorders. In general, females are more likely than males to binge eat, use extreme weight control practices (skipping meals, fasting, self-inducing vomiting, misusing

TEXT BOX 2.1

Anorexia nervosa in Curacao

Anorexia nervosa is believed to be much more common in affluent and westernized cultures that value thinness as an ideal body image. Research has shown that eating disorders exist in many countries throughout the world and that anorexia nervosa emerges in countries undergoing modernization and westernization. Hans Hoek and his colleagues (Hoek, van Harten, Hermans, Katzman, Matroos, & Susser, 2005; Katzman, Hermans, van Hoeken, & Hoek, 2004) performed an exhaustive study of the incidence of anorexia nervosa in Curacao, a Caribbean island undergoing socioeconomic transition.

Hoek et al. (2005) contacted all community health and clinical service providers and all 82 general practitioners on the island as well as reviewed inpatient records for 84,420 hospital admissions to the three hospitals between 1995 and 1998. They identified probable cases of anorexia nervosa from these sources and then interviewed them. While the overall incidence of anorexia nervosa on Curacao was lower than found in similar studies in the United States and the Netherlands, a markedly discrepant pattern was observed by ethnicity. No cases of anorexia nervosa were found in the majority black population in Curacao. In contrast, the incidence rate among the minority groups in Curacao (mixed race and white population) were similar to that of the United States and the Netherlands. This study provides impressive support for the view that sociocultural factors are associated with different rates of anorexia nervosa.

Katzman et al. (2004) conducted a detailed study of cases of anorexia nervosa in Curacao using interviews and questionnaires. To obtain a broader context, they also assessed matched controls. The women with anorexia nervosa were "not your typical island woman" (p. 463). None of the women with AN were black. The women with anorexia nervosa were highly educated, wealthy, and had traveled extensively overseas. Psychologically, the women with anorexia nervosa were more perfectionistic and anxious than the control women. The women with anorexia nervosa viewed themselves as different from the cultural norm and from the majority group of black women. Katzman and colleagues (2004) noted that these women were experiencing three challenges to their identity. First, they were mixed race and aspiring to fit into the upwardly mobile and mostly white subculture while distancing themselves from the black majority. Second, they had extensive education and travel which produced conflicts between modern and traditional views of being a female. Third, travel oversees made living within the island culture frustrating because of perceived limitations.

laxatives, diuretics, and diet pills), and to have greater body image dissatisfaction (Barry & Grilo, 2002; Cash et al., 2004; Grunbaum et al., 2004). This gender disparity is found across all age and developmental eras. In general, Caucasians are more likely to use extreme weight control practices and to have greater body image concerns than other ethnic minority groups (Akan & Grilo, 1995; Cash et al., 2004; Neumark-Sztainer et al., 2002a). Research in recent years has generally supported these overall findings by gender and ethnicity but has revealed that such problems are not uncommon in males or ethnic minorities and must not be overlooked.

Epidemiology and distribution of obesity

Obesity in the United States

In contrast to the eating disorders, obesity has been studied in large epidemiological studies. In the United States, the most recent findings from the National Health and Nutrition Examination Survey (NHANES, 2001–2) indicate that 66% of the adult population is overweight and 31% is obese (Hedley et al., 2004). Compared to the 1999–2000 period, the prevalence of severe obesity (BMI = 40.0) increased to 5.1% (Hedley et al., 2004). This translates to over 34 million obese individuals in the United States. Large-scale research has shown convincingly that the prevalence of obesity has been rising steadily (Hedley et al., 2004; Kuczmarski, Flegal, Campbell, & Johnson, 1994). Figure 2.3 summarizes the most recent estimates of overweight and obesity separately by gender and ethnicity for the US. As is evident from Figure 2.3, in the US, obesity is common in both men and women, with higher rates in women, and is especially common in certain ethnic minority groups (particularly hispanic and black groups). Interestingly, self-perception of obesity tends to be more common in women than men and in whites compared with black and hispanic groups (Paeratakul, White, Williamson, Ryan, &

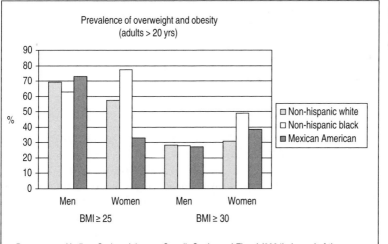

Prevalence of overweight and obesity
(adults > 20 yrs)

Legend:
- Non-hispanic white
- Non-hispanic black
- Mexican American

Men / Women — BMI ≥ 25
Men / Women — BMI ≥ 30

Data source: Hedley, Ogden, Johnson, Carroll, Curtin, and Flegal (2004) *Journal of the American Medical Association.*

Figure 2.3.
Increasing prevalence of obesity.

Bray, 2002). In the US, a higher distribution of obesity is associated with (in addition to gender and ethnicity) older age, lower socio-economic status, marital status, and (if female) multiparous.

Obesity worldwide

Worldwide, there is clear evidence for the increasing prevalence of obesity, which is now universally regarded as one of the world's major health problems (World Health Organization, 1992, 1998). What is particularly striking is the marked disparities in obesity rates across different countries worldwide. Interestingly, there are marked disparities in obesity across different countries within regions (e.g., within Europe there are wide variations as well as within Africa). Marked disparities in obesity rates exist across both modernized and developing countries. Consider the following prevalence rates reported by the WHO (1998). China has one of the lowest prevalence rates in the world, recently estimated to be 0.4% of men and 0.9% of women. Japan, a highly modernized country, has an estimated obesity prevalence of 2% of men and 3% of women. Within Europe, much variation exists; the prevalence of obesity in England (15% of men and 17% of women), for example, is much higher than in Sweden (5% of men and 9% of women). Within the Middle East, the prevalence of obesity in Kuwait (32% of men and 44% of women) is twice that in Saudi Arabia (16% of men and 24% of women). At the other end of the spectrum, the prevalence of obesity in urban Samoa is 58% of men and 77% of women. Worldwide, a higher distribution of obesity is associated with older age, female, lower socioeconomic status, marital status, and (if female) with multiple pregnancies.

Overweight and obesity in children and adolescents

Although there is no universally adopted definition of obesity for children (Cole, Bellizzi, Flegal, & Dietz, 2000; Troiano & Flegal, 1999) as there is for adults (chapter 1), inspection of weight data and comparison to various reference curves for weight by age clearly suggests a dramatic increase in overweight in children during the past 20 years (Ogden, Troiano, Briefel, Kuczmarski, Flegal, & Johnson, 1997; Troiano & Flegal, 1999). Roughly 11% of children aged 6 to 17 have BMIs estimated to be above the 95th percentile. Roughly 15% of adolescents are considered obese (95th percentile) and an additional 22% (85th–95th percentile) are considered overweight. Among younger persons, roughly 11% of girls aged 4 to 5 are now considered to be overweight. These prevalence estimates reflect two- to three-fold increases during the past 20 years.

Development and course of eating disorders

Anorexia nervosa

Anorexia nervosa most typically begins in adolescence. The onset of AN typically follows a period of restrictive dieting which is sometimes triggered by stressful life events or transitions. Although dieting behaviors are nearly universal in adolescents and the majority have body image concerns (Neumark-Sztainer, Story, Hannan, Perry, & Irving, 2002b) only a very small portion go on to develop AN or BN. For reasons that are not understood, the dietary restriction intensifies in susceptible persons and soon takes over the person's life. Initially, these individuals are reinforced by the weight loss. Soon the dietary restriction and control over eating provide a sense of control or mastery over the body, which represents an escape from uncertainty and distress about life's circumstances.

The course (i.e., the temporal pattern over time) and outcome (i.e., specific state at some particular time) of AN are highly variable across individuals. In some cases, this problem develops only partially or even fully only to be short-lived and to resolve without many biopsychosocial consequences (described later in chapter 3). In other cases, AN develops into a highly resistant, chronic, and life-threatening problem. In such cases, the dietary restriction continues to intensify and fuel perfectionistic and obsessional styles characteristic of many of these individuals. A vicious self-perpetuating spiral serves to maintain the disorder. With increasing weight loss, the fear of fatness and the overevaluation of shape and weight seem to intensify as the perfectionistic standards regarding eating or weight become increasingly difficult to attain, resulting in turn in greater restriction and other weight control behaviors (e.g., excessive exercise). At the same time, the importance of the perceived control grows and the increased restriction and weight loss are seen as signs of success, rather than reflecting a dangerous disorder. It is also not uncommon for individuals with AN to alternate between periods of tight dietary restriction (with or without excessive exercise) and periods of binge eating and purging at different points in the course of their illness (Casper et al., 1980; Eckert et al., 1995; Eddy et al., 2002). Over time, up to half of patients with AN eventually develop binge eating (Eddy et al., 2002) and full criteria for BN (Bulik et al., 1997b).

Even with intensive treatment, studies generally find that fewer than 50% of patients with AN recover, roughly one-third improve, and 20% show a chronic and disabling life course (Steinhausen, 2002; Zipfel, Lowe, Reas, Deter, & Herzog, 2000). Carefully conducted prospective longitudinal studies of AN have documented high rates of symptom persistence and only partial recovery in many patients (Fichter & Quadflieg, 1997; Herzog et al., 1999; Strober, Freeman, & Morrell, 1997). Even among AN patients who appear to achieve a full recovery, roughly one-third relapse (Herzog et al., 1999; Strober et al., 1997). Among patients who no longer meet criteria for AN, lifelong struggles continue with relatively low weight and substantial body image psychopathology as well as with certain psychological features (e.g., perfectionism and obsessiveness) that often persist despite some improvement in the AN itself (Sullivan, Bulik, Fear, & Pickering, 1998). Follow-up studies of patients with AN also find high rates of additional psychiatric disorders (Steinhausen, 2002). Very high rates of depression, anxiety, and alcohol use disorders are found in patients with AN over their life course (Sullivan et al., 1998). AN is associated with substantially elevated mortality (Crisp, Callender, Halek, & Hsu, 1992; Keel, Dorer, Eddy, Franko, Charatan, & Herzog, 2003), which is estimated at 5.6% per decade (Sullivan, 1995). Eating disorders, along with substance use disorders, have the highest mortality rates of all psychiatric disorders (Keel et al., 2003). Most deaths result from starvation, cardiac events, or suicide.

Predicting course and outcome in AN is difficult, but a few general predictors have been identified (Herpertz-Dahlmann, Muller, Herpertz, Heussen, Hebebrand, & Remschmidt, 2001; Keel et al., 2003; Steinhausen, 2002). In general, earlier age of onset, short history of illness, and limited weight loss are good prognostic indicators. Longer duration of illness, severe weight loss and low weight, binge eating and vomiting, and high psychiatric co-morbidity are associated with poor prognosis. Alcohol use disorders have been identified as a predictor of elevated mortality among patients with AN (Keel et al., 2003).

Bulimia nervosa

Bulimia nervosa most typically begins in late adolescence and early adulthood. Like AN, the onset of BN frequently follows a period of restrictive dieting, including some cases in which the course of AN develops or evolves into BN (Bulik et al., 1997b; Tozzi et al., 2005). As the dietary restriction intensifies individuals begin to experience episodes of uncontrolled overeating or binge eating. Binge eating is well known to occur after periods of restrictive dieting. Indeed, the classic semi-starvation diet of normal healthy volunteers demonstrated this (Keys, Brozek, Henschel, Mickelson, & Taylor, 1950). The restrictive dieting results in both physiological and psychological deprivation and is readily disrupted by numerous factors (e.g., negative emotional states, stressful events, food cues, alcohol, etc.). Again, for uncertain reasons, the binge eating begins to occur with increasing frequency in susceptible persons who do not lessen their attempts at dieting restrictively. These episodes of binge eating intensify concerns regarding shape and weight and soon individuals begin to use extreme weight control and purging behaviors such as self-inducing vomiting after binge eating. Soon, these behaviors spiral out of control in susceptible persons. Once developed, BN is a self-maintaining vicious cycle:

1   Restrictive dieting and deprivation triggers binge eating or the dietary control is interrupted by internal/external factors resulting in binge eating.
2   The binge eating results in physical and emotional distress including fear of weight gain.
3   The binge sequelae trigger purging or other extreme weight control practices to undo the caloric intake and emotional fear of weight gain.
4   The purging is followed by shame and disgust.
5   The core cognitive features (overevaluation of shape and weight) are both intensified by these behaviors as well as lead to attempts at re-establishing dietary control.
6   These heightened concerns and the overly restrictive dieting set the stage for repeating the BN cycle.

The course and outcome of BN are, like the case for AN, highly variable across individuals. The course and outcome of BN, however, are consistently more positive than that of AN. In one of the methodologically strongest longitudinal studies, Herzog and colleagues (1999) reported that the recovery rate for BN was 74% (versus only 33% for AN) by 90 months of follow-up. In general, in some cases, BN develops only partially or can develop fully only to be short-lived and to resolve for uncertain reasons or as the result of certain treatments (Wilson, 2005). In many other instances, BN develops into a serious problem that can take on a chronic course (Keel & Mitchell, 1997; Quadflieg & Fichter, 2003). Long-term follow-up studies have found, for example, that roughly 30% of BN patients still experience significant problems with binge eating and vomiting even after ten years (Keel, Mitchell, Miller, Davis, & Crow, 1999). Fairburn and colleagues (2000), in a follow-up study of a community-based sample of persons with BN, also reported a relatively poor prognosis. At each assessment point, between half and two-thirds of BN patients continued to experience significant symptoms although many were slightly below the level required for BN diagnosis. A variable fluctuating pattern over time was observed with each year roughly a third showing improvement and a third relapsing (Fairburn et al., 2000). In contrast to the high rates of diagnostic crossover from AN to BN over time (Bulik et al., 1997b), few cases of BN cross over into AN over time (Fichter & Quadflieg, 2004; Keel et al., 1999). BN is associated with substantially elevated psychiatric morbidity with elevated rates of depression, anxiety, and substance use disorders most commonly observed (Fichter & Quadflieg, 2004). In contrast to AN, BN, is not associated with significantly elevated rates of mortality (Keel et al., 2003).

Predicting course and outcome in BN has proven to be very difficult. Although there are isolated findings that certain factors such as psychiatric co-morbidity may be a negative prognostic indictor (Fichter & Quadflieg, 2004; Keel et al., 1999) most studies have failed to find predictors of outcomes (Herzog et al., 1999). In general, reliable predictors of outcome for BN have not been identified.

Binge eating disorder and eating disorder not otherwise specified

Very little is known about the development and course of BED and EDNOS. Clinical observations suggest that both develop following various dieting attempts and spiral out of control in susceptible persons. EDNOS is likely to be found across all developmental eras and to often begin in adolescence. In contrast, BED is thought to have a much later average age at onset than either AN and BN. Most treatment studies, for example, retrospectively trace back the onset of the BED to an average age in the early to mid-twenties. Interestingly, and in sharp contrast to AN and BN, several research studies have found that up to half of patients with BED report that they began to binge eat *prior* to their first diet (Grilo & Masheb, 2000; Mussell, Mitchell, Weller, Raymond, Crow, & Crosby, 1995; Spurrell, Wilfley,

Tanofsky, & Brownell, 1997). These studies have found relatively few differences between patients who reported dieting first versus binge eating first and highlight the possibility of binge eating as a risk factor for subsequent obesity.

Even less is known about the course and outcome of BED and EDNOS. Retrospective clinical accounts from persons with BED suggest longstanding histories although many patients seem to have periods that are symptom free and other periods of fluctuating symptoms. Two studies of the natural course of BED suggest moderate rates of symptom remissions over time (Cachelin, Striegel-Moore, Elder, Pike, Wilfley, & Fairburn, 1999; Fairburn et al., 2000) while a more recent six-year study reported a poorer pattern of outcome (Fichter, 2005; Fichter et al., 2003). Fairburn and colleagues (2000), in a community-based five-year naturalistic study, reported that the outcome of BED was significantly better than that for BN and that there was little diagnostic crossover. The BED cohort in this study was significantly younger and had had a much lower BMI than BED patients in most clinical studies. Importantly, BED patients in this study were found to gain weight throughout the study and the rate of obesity increased from 21% to 39% during the five-year period. Fichter (2005) recently reported the six-year course of patients with BED was characterized by moderate levels of continued disturbed eating and psychosocial problems that were comparable or slightly worse than those in patients with BN. Three studies of the natural course and outcome of patients with EDNOS reported moderately persistent problems over time (Grilo et al., 2003a; Herzog et al., 1993; Milos, Spindler, Schnyder, & Fairburn, 2005). Grilo and colleagues (2003a) reported a remission rate of 59% for EDNOS versus 40% for BN over a 24-month period and that psychiatric and personality disorder co-morbidity did not predict course.

Development and course of obesity

Overweight and obesity develop throughout the lifespan. As noted above, in many countries worldwide, the prevalence of obesity is increasing. The increasing prevalence of obesity in children and adolescents is particularly alarming. Epidemiological research clearly suggests a dramatic increase in overweight in children during the past 20 years (Ogden et al., 1997). Thus, people are increasingly developing obesity at an earlier age. Research has suggested that childhood overweight is not merely a passing or fleeting problem but instead represents a pressing health concern for reasons noted below.

First, childhood obesity frequently persists or tracks into adulthood. It has been estimated that 80% of overweight adolescents become obese adults (Casey, Dwyer, Coleman, & Valadian, 1992; Garn, Sullivan, & Hawthorne, 1989). Recent research has improved the precision with which adult obesity can be predicted from childhood and adolescent weight (Bray, 2002; Guo, Wu, Chumlea, & Roche, 2002). Guo and colleagues (2002) developed formulas to identify obese adults using data from the Fels Longitudinal Study. For example, for girls at the 95th percentile of BMI, the probability of becoming obese adults was between 40% and 60% from ages 5 to 12 and this rise increased further after age 12. Bray (2002a) notes a number of additional risk factors that been identified for predicting adult obesity. For example, children whose mothers developed gestational diabetes had higher rates of obesity in adulthood as did children of mothers who smoked during pregnancy despite their lower birth weights (e.g., Power & Jefferis, 2002).

Second, childhood obesity is associated with high medical risks throughout the lifespan. Adolescents who are obese suffer from high rates of medical problems as adults (DiPietro, Mossberg, & Stunkard, 1994). Moreover, overweight children appear to be at high risk for developing health problems at an early age. In particular, type II diabetes in children is increasing rapidly and seems commensurate with the increase in obesity (Pinhas-Hamiel, Dolan, Daniels, Standiford, Khoury, & Zeitler, 1996). The course of obesity is generally regarded as chronic. Although many obese persons lose weight on their own or with professional programs (chapter 6), most typically regain most of the weight back within five years. Hence, over the lifespan through the fifties, the general pattern is a continued increase in excess weight with episodic fluctuations of periods of weight loss.

Possible etiological and risk factors for eating disorders

The etiology of the eating disorders (anorexia nervosa and bulimia nervosa) is largely unknown. There is some consensus that environmental factors, including potent sociocultural pressures to achieve certain body ideals, play an important role in the development of eating disorders. It is likely, however, that eating disorders have complex multi-factorial causes. Thus, in addition to the sociocultural factors and context, there likely exist complex and multiple forms of interplay among genetic, familial and non-familial environments, psychological factors, and temperamental factors. By interplay it is suggested that the influences can be multiple and varied in direction. For example, consider that while a certain environmental factor or pressure (e.g., achieve thin ideal) may have its influence felt more strongly by a susceptible person (e.g., someone with genetic and/or psychological vulnerabilities), someone with that profile may also more actively seek out certain environments characterized by those pressures (e.g., someone with an "anorexia makeup" may pursue an aesthetically demanding field such as ballet).

Unrealistic body image ideals

Idealized body images have probably changed in recent times. The "plumpness" or "fullness" emphasized by artists in their works through the eighteenth centuries have been replaced, in westernized and developed societies by ideals emphasizing leanness. The twentieth-century ideals of thinness have differed markedly in the explosion of media and communication methods. This is one major reason that the eating disorders can perhaps be thought of as "modern" disorders (Vandereycken, 2002). Indeed, unrealistic body shape and body weight ideals are portrayed everywhere. Western society's pervasive emphasis on thinness as the ideal is portrayed throughout every media in seemingly endless ways. An example of the longstanding portrayal of body weight and shape in westernized countries can be found in two selected examples of "ideal" female body images. Figure 2.4 summarizes the average BMI for Miss America Contestant winners and for *Playboy* centerfolds recorded decade by decade. As shown in the figure, since the 1930s, the average BMI of these women has been below 19.5. Indeed, the average BMI for the 1970s through 1990s was below 19.

Children are also constantly exposed to similar unrealistic ideals regarding weight and shape. Brownell and Napolitanio (1995) examined the body proportions in two very popular dolls in the United States (Barbie and Ken) to determine the extent to which they vary from the actual proportions of young healthy women and men. The authors took measurements (chest, waist, etc.) of a 22-year-old female who was 5 feet 2 inches tall and weighed 125 pounds and of a 32-year-old male who was 6 feet tall and weighed 185 pounds. Figure 2.5 shows the percentage change in the actual measurements of two

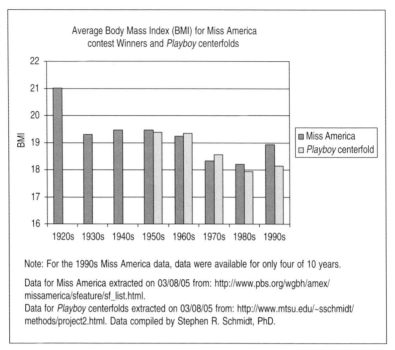

Figure 2.4.
Selected societal "ideal" female body images over time.

Average Body Mass Index (BMI) for Miss America contest Winners and *Playboy* centerfolds

Note: For the 1990s Miss America data, data were available for only four of 10 years.

Data for Miss America extracted on 03/08/05 from: http://www.pbs.org/wgbh/amex/missamerica/sfeature/sf_list.html.
Data for *Playboy* centerfolds extracted on 03/08/05 from: http://www.mtsu.edu/~sschmidt/methods/project2.html. Data compiled by Stephen R. Schmidt, PhD.

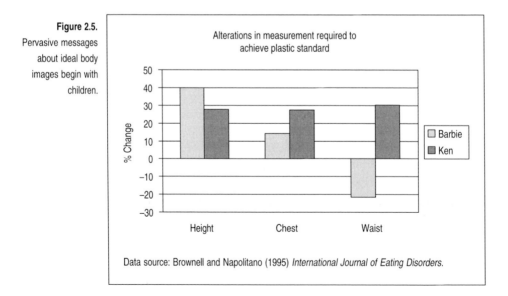

Figure 2.5.
Pervasive messages about ideal body images begin with children.

Alterations in measurement required to achieve plastic standard

Data source: Brownell and Napolitano (1995) *International Journal of Eating Disorders*.

healthy young adults that would be required to fit the proportions of the Barbie and Ken dolls (the plastic standard of ideal bodies for children). As shown in Figure 2.5, the woman would need to be 40% taller, increase her chest measurement by 15%, and decrease her waist measurement by 22%. The man would need to be 29% taller, increase his chest by 28%, and increase his waist by 30%. The authors concluded that young children, like adults, are exposed to highly unrealistic ideals of shape and weight.

Who is vulnerable? Etiology and risk factors

The obvious question is why do only a small percentage of people, and most frequently girls and women, go on to develop eating disorders? These pervasive images contribute to widespread discontent, stigma, and biases while producing incredible economic benefits for those who market many diverse products. These pervasive images, however, only result in eating disorders in relatively few people – i.e., those who are somehow susceptible. There is probably a complex genetic risk and there are likely a range of diverse environmental risk factors that combine in ways that are still unknown (Becker, Keel, Anderson-Fye, & Thomas, 2004). A general schematic of genetic risks and environmental factors and their interplay with psychological and temperamental features is shown in Text Box 2.2.

As with many psychiatric and medical disorders, there is evidence that there are genetic and familial components to eating disorders (Becker et al., 2004; Bulik & Tozzi, 2004; Klump & Gobrogge, 2005; Lilenfeld et al., 1998; Strober, Freeman, Lampert, Diamond, & Kaye, 2000). Studies have suggested shared familial liability to eating disorders, with some possible degree of cross-transmission between AN, BN, and other forms of eating problems. Several things complicate research in this area. Other psychiatric problems frequently co-existing with eating disorders also seem to run in families in complicated patterns. Research has also found increased rates of alcohol problems in family members of patients with BN but no evidence for cross-transmission (Kaye et al., 1996). Some studies have noted an increased rate of depression in family members of patients with eating disorders and although there may be some shared genetic and environmental risks for anorexia nervosa and depression (Wade et al., 2000). Perhaps a bigger challenge is there remain questions about how best to define eating disorders and what is the exact nature of their underlying features. These complexities notwithstanding,

TEXT BOX 2.2

Overview of general etiological model of eating disorders

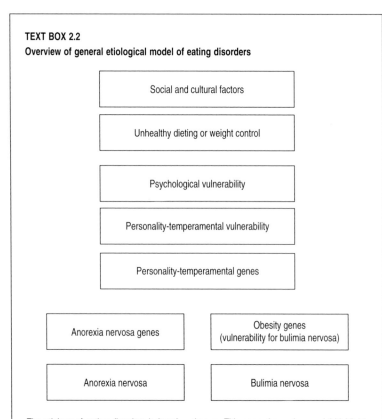

The etiology of eating disorders is largely unknown. This general overview model highlights general factors that are thought to play some etiological role in the development of eating disorders. There are probably complex and multiple forms of interplay among these factors. Hence, the diagram is intended to suggest a dynamic system rather than a simply sequence. Sociocultural pressures to attain certain physical ideals are pervasive and are necessary influences for the development of eating disorders. Unhealthy dieting or weight control attempts generally precede full-blown eating disorders. Only some people develop unhealthy patterns and only a small percentage of those who engage in unhealthy dieting/weight control behaviors (i.e., problems) develop eating disorders (i.e., clinical disorders). There must be certain vulnerabilities that make some people especially susceptible to those pressures and to other environmental (familial and non-familial) factors.

Although there may be common influences (sociocultural pressures and unhealthy dieting or weight control) and risk factors (female gender, psychological vulnerabilities such as poor self-esteem) to all eating disorders, anorexia nervosa and bulimia nervosa may be distinct disorders reflecting different biological and temperamental vulnerabilities. Indeed, there exist tempera-mental differences between anorexia nervosa (obsessiveness, rigidity/inflexibility, perfectionism, harm avoidance) and bulimia nervosa (novelty seeking, impulsivity). These differences converge with findings from molecular genetic research suggesting anorexia nervosa and bulimia nervosa have distinctly different underlying biological (genetic) vulnerabilities.

eating disorders do appear to have some familial transmission that increases vulnerability or likelihood of developing a problem.

The available twin studies generally report much higher concordance rates for monozygotic (MZ) twins (50% for AN and 30% for BN) than for dizygotic (DZ) twins (5% to 10%). MZ twins are genetically identical and share 100% of their genetic information whereas DZ twins share on average 50% of their genetic information (like any other sibling pair). Thus, the higher rate in MZ than DZ twins suggests a genetic effect particularly since MZ and DZ twins are the same age and reared by parents at the same time. One recent review of the available genetic studies concluded that the magnitude of the genetic contribution to the eating disorders is uncertain given the wide variation in estimates across studies and the limitations in the research conducted to date (Fairburn & Harrison, 2003). A more circumspect stance, however, is that there is a significant genetic contribution to both AN and BN as well as more broadly to their components, and this seems to be the emerging consensus (Bulik et al., 2000b; Collier & Treasure, 2005; Klump & Gobrogge, 2005). There are no adoption studies of eating disorders, which would provide critically important additional information about genetic factors and aspects of the rearing environment.

The findings suggesting the importance of genetic factors have fueled more sophisticated genetic studies. In particular, recent years have witnessed aggressive interest in molecular genetic research on eating disorders and associated traits. Recent reviews of the emerging findings from molecular genetic research attempting to identify susceptibility genes suggest some trends (Collier & Treasure, 2005; Klump and Gobrogge, 2005), although replication of findings is difficult and much uncertainty remains.

Molecular genetics research falls into two categories. Association studies compare eating disorder patients to control patients without the eating disorder and are utilized when there are "candidate" genes based on theory or prior research (Tozzi & Bulik, 2003). Linkage studies refer to exploratory studies (with fewer hypotheses) and involve studying families with at least one person affected with an eating disorder. Linkage studies analyze whether family members with the same disorder share any markers on chromosome regions (rather than specific genes) at greater than chance levels. Linkage studies have suggested the possible involvement of anorexia nervosa (but not bulimia nervosa) to chromosome 1 (Grice et al., 2002). Bulik and colleagues (2003) linked purging types of bulimia nervosa to chromosome 10. The positive finding for chromosome 10 in bulimia nervosa, which has also been linked to obesity (Hager et al., 1998), is consistent with risk factor studies (Fairburn, Doll, Welch, Hay, Davies, & O'Connor, 1998) reporting greater familial obesity in bulimia nervosa than in anorexia nervosa.

Particularly relevant to genetic approaches is research consistently documenting the importance of certain temperamental or personality traits. Persons who are perfectionistic, obsessional, and rigid and who are behaviorally characterized as harm avoidant or fearful tend to appear to be especially vulnerable to falling victim to anorexia nervosa following restrictive dieting. In people with these temperamental or personality styles, the highly restrictive dieting provides an important sense of control or mastery while the initial weight loss is rewarding since it partly addresses some of the overevaluation of shape and weight concerns. In contrast, people who are characterized by a novelty-seeking type of temperament and who are impulsive appear to be more susceptible to developing bulimia nervosa (rather than anorexia nervosa) following the restrictive dieting.

Accordingly, research examining both genetic and environmental contributions to eating disorders has broadened to include such temperamental and personality traits in addition to the eating disorder features (Anderluh et al., 2003; Bulik et al., 2005; Devlin et al., 2002). Obsessiveness, rigidity, and perfectionism seem to aggregate in families of patients with AN (Lilenfeld et al., 1998). Some of these traits persist even after recovery or improvement from the eating disorder (Lilenfeld et al., 2000; Tchanturia et al., 2004). Importantly, Devlin and colleagues (2002) reported analyses suggested that obsessionality is associated with chromosome 1, which has been linked to anorexia nervosa. These temperamental differences between anorexia nervosa and bulimia nervosa converge with emerging findings from molecular genetic research suggesting anorexia nervosa (Devlin et al., 2002) and bulimia nervosa (Bulik et al., 2003) have distinctly different underlying biological vulnerabilities (Collier & Treasure, 2004). Thus, although there may be common risk factors to all eating disorders, anorexia nervosa and bulimia nervosa may be distinct disorders reflecting different biological and temperamental vulnerabilities.

In contrast to the relatively little research on the genetics of eating disorders (although that field is rapidly growing) is the large volume of research on risk factors for eating disorders. Although a variety of risk factors have been posited, firm evidence has not yet been found for any of these, except for: female gender, developmental time frame of adolescence through early adulthood, and westernized society or ideals. There is a fair amount of empirical support for a number of familial factors, including: an eating disorder, depressive disorders, and – more specifically for bulimia – alcohol use problems and familial obesity (Fairburn, Welch, Doll, & Davies, 1997; Fairburn et al. 1998). In terms of environmental factors, it is critical to consider non-familial (not shared by family members) influences (Klump, Wonderlich, Lehoux, Lilenfeld, & Bulik, 2002) in addition to family factors. In terms of environmental influences, several adverse experiences have received some support as potential factors, including: chaotic and negative familial and caregiving environment, childhood maltreatment, negative or critical commentary or teasing about shape or weight, familial overconcern with dieting, peer influences to diet, peer or performance pressures (e.g., ballet performance given the extreme aesthetic requirements, other sports with weight requirements). In terms of psychological factors, it is generally thought that persons who have low self-esteem plus have a heightened interpersonal sensitivity along with social deficits may be especially vulnerable to the pervasive sociocultural pressures to attain a certain body shape ideal.

The etiology and maintenance of obesity

Obesity is a complex and very heterogeneous disorder (Brownell & Wadden, 1991, 1992) that has sometimes been referred to as "obesities" to reflect both its multi-factorial nature and its various forms. With that said, most forms of obesity reflect complex biopsychosocial factors and these factors may vary substantially over time. The contributing factors may vary over time within individuals over their lifespan and may vary over time across individuals given substantive environmental shits (e.g., famine or abundance). It is important to consider the current worldwide epidemic of obesity when attempting to grasp the nature of the various potential contributors to obesity.

Obesity and positive energy balance result from complex genetic and environmental influences (Grilo & Pogue-Geile, 1991) that are still not well understood. At the simplest level, obesity results from energy imbalance, i.e., fat develops from taking in more calories than are used for energy. For many decades, the average adult gained one pound per year. Thus, on average an average 40-year-old would weigh 20 pounds more than they did at age 20. The remarkable thing about this general statement is that the human body must posses a highly efficient energy regulation system to make this happen. Consider how many meals are eaten every year and how variable those meals and snacks can be from day to day. Consider also how variable lifestyle physical activity and exercise habits can be from week to week. Consider also how variable things like illnesses, weather, and vacations can be since these factors also influence energy intake and expenditure. When these factors are considered, the average weight change of one pound per year takes on a different meaning. Indeed, it suggests that the human body possesses elaborate systems of energy regulation.

Indeed, considerable research has demonstrated the human body's adaptations to overfeeding and underfeeding in various permutations. At the simplest level, underfeeding (caloric restriction) results in decreased energy expenditure (e.g., a drop in resting metabolic rate). This physiologic adaptation is one reason for the sometimes observed slowing of weight loss during dieting (Grilo, Brownell, & Stunkard, 1993). Less impressive, but certainly measurable, is the increased resting metabolic rates in response to overeating. The remarkable increase in the prevalence of obesity in children, adolescents, and adults during the past two decades suggests that environmental shifts have been able to override the physiological mechanisms responsible for energy balance.

While there are many possible contributing factors and complex combinations of factors, at the simplest level, obesity results from eating more calories than are burned off (i.e., the first law of thermodynamics). It is also important to emphasize that although the current epidemic of obesity is perhaps fueled by environmental shifts, this does not mean that genetics and biology are unimportant for these probably influence the degree of susceptibility or vulnerability to the environmental shifts. Indeed, while the first law of thermodynamics accounts for the outcome (obesity), it does not describe the complex molecular (genetic), physiological, and behavioral pathways that regulate intake and expenditure (Bray & Champagne, 2005). As Bray and Champagne (2005) noted, "there is more to obesity than kilocalories" (p. 17).

With these general principles in mind, a few examples of likely contributors to obesity will be highlighted. These examples were chosen because of their importance and to raise critical issues; these examples do not by any means represent an exhaustive listing. There exist many other factors, some with compelling research support, which are likely to play important roles in the development of obesity, both in individuals as well as at the societal level (Keith et al., in press). There are also many important factors (gender, age, ethnicity, and so forth) that influence energy balance between groups as well as over time (DeLany, Bray, Harsha, & Volaufova, 2002). The first few examples reflect factors that very likely account for increasing obesity within individuals over time as well as for the increasing prevalence of obesity in our society. The two factors are increased caloric intake (specifically increased portion size and increased consumption of fast food) and decreased physical activity.

Eating too much

Common sense and the first law of thermodynamics tell us that eating too many calories and too much fat will result in obesity. The preponderance of research with animals and humans supports this. A seemingly endless array of popular diet books and plans effectively marketed across all media outlets touting a plethora of dietary plans (along with outlandish claims of unsubstantiated success and promises of easy and longstanding weight loss) seems to have overpowered both common sense and scientific knowledge. To reduce the facts to the simplest level: if a person eats more calories than they burn off then they will gain weight and fat. As already noted above, there is considerable variation across people in their susceptibility to gain weight and fat in response to overeating calories and overeating dietary fat. Nonetheless, on average, persons who eat more total calories and who eat a diet comprised of a greater amount of dietary fat will be substantially more likely to become obese than those who eat fewer calories and less fat (Bray & Popkin, 1998).

Willet (1998), in a review of epidemiological and clinical studies, noted a weak association between total fat intake and obesity and raised the provocative question whether high dietary fat diets are a cause of obesity. A major problem with this perspective is the insufficient attention paid to total caloric intake in addition to dietary fat intake. Indeed, Bray and Popkin (1998, 1999), in a review of literature, including a critical review of 28 clinical trials, concluded that reductions in dietary fat (and proportion of energy from fat) was associated with weight loss. Experimental studies with laboratory animals that allow for careful control of many potential factors have clearly demonstrated these basic findings, i.e., that both caloric intake and dietary fat intake are important for determining obesity (Petro et al., 2004).

Increased portion sizes

Meals with larger portion sizes will, on average, have more calories. Of course, this is not necessarily always the case. It is possible, for example, to have large portions of low caloric foods (e.g., certain large salads without high fat dressings or toppings). By and large, however, bigger portions generally do result in more calories. A recent study (Diliberti, Bordi, Conklin, Roe, & Rolls, 2004) systematically altered the size of a pasta entrée on different days from a standard portion (248 g) to a large portion (377 g) without a price change. Diners who purchased the larger portion increased their total eating of the entrée by 43% (172 kcal) and of the entire meal by 25% (159 kcal). Hence, being offered or served a larger portion sets the stage for excess eating and generally results in overeating.

Do larger portion sizes really matter?

It can be argued that serving larger portions does not necessarily cause overeating. Intuitively, one would predict that if a person is not hungry or if the food is not appealing, they will not overeat. A series of controlled experiments, however, have produced impressive evidence demonstrating the overriding impact of serving sizes on eating behaviors. One study found that larger serving bowls at a superbowl party led to 56% greater food intake (Wansink & Cheney, 2005). Another controlled experimental study compared eating by persons attending a movie who were randomly given either a medium or a large container of free popcorn that was either fresh or stale (Wansink & Kim, 2005). Persons who were given fresh popcorn ate 45.3% more popcorn when it was provided in a large container. Amazingly, even when the popcorn provided was stale, subjects ate 33.6% more when it was from a large container. These studies suggest that large food containers or servings can lead to overeating and can even override taste. The interested reader is referred to the recent review by Wansink (2004) on a range of environmental factors (e.g., package size, plate shape, lighting, etc.) that have been demonstrated to influence eating behaviors. It seems that there are many such factors (well known to food manufacturers and marketers but not recognized by consumers) that influence eating. These factors generally work by inhibiting or decreasing how much we pay attention while providing cues that suggest different eating norms (e.g., this is a serving). It is important to emphasize that such shifts in portion size and food containers are likely to impact greatly on children. Research has demonstrated that children also regulate their eating poorly and rely greatly on what adults serve them and are especially responsive to environmental cues (Mrdjenovic & Levitsky, 2005).

A recent experiment attempted to further disentangle the potential roles of visual cues (portion sizes) and internal states such as hunger and awareness of eating. In a classic study entitled the "bottomless bowls," Wansink, Painter, and North (2005) tested whether visual cues of portion size can influence how much people eat without changing how much they think they eat or how full they feel. Fifty-four subjects of varying weight participated in a study of "eating a soup-only lunch and completing a questionnaire." The subjects were either provided soup in a normal bowl or were provided soup in a bowl that looked the same but was rigged as a self-refilling bowl (to prove a biased visual cue). The results are summarized in Figure 2.6. Subjects who unknowingly ate from the self-refilling bowl ate 73% more food (14.7 ounces versus 8.5 ounces, which translated to 268 calories versus 155 calories) than subjects who ate from the same

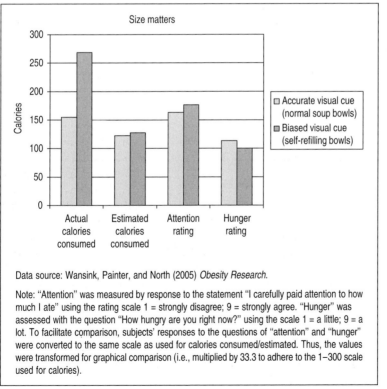

Data source: Wansink, Painter, and North (2005) *Obesity Research.*

Note: "Attention" was measured by response to the statement "I carefully paid attention to how much I ate" using the rating scale 1 = strongly disagree; 9 = strongly agree. "Hunger" was assessed with the question "How hungry are you right now?" using the scale 1 = a little; 9 = a lot. To facilitate comparison, subjects' responses to the questions of "attention" and "hunger" were converted to the same scale as used for calories consumed/estimated. Thus, the values were transformed for graphical comparison (i.e., multiplied by 33.3 to adhere to the 1–300 scale used for calories).

Figure 2.6.
Does portion or serving size of food matter?

bowl that did not refill itself. Despite eating 73% more soup, the subjects who ate from the "bottomless bowl" did not think that they ate more than those subjects who ate from the regular bowls. Interestingly, these subjects ate significantly more despite similar ratings of hunger and how much attention they paid to food.

Portion size increases parallel increases in obesity

There is compelling evidence that the rising prevalence of obesity during the past few decades has been paralleled by increases in the portion sizes of many foods and by the frequency of eating fast foods (i.e., high fat and densely high caloric foods) away from home. Figure 2.7 summarizes data reported by Nielsen and Popkin (2003) and Astrup (2005) showing the percentage of changes in kcal contained in the increasing portion sizes of popular foods from 1977–78 to 1994–96. As can be seen, for example, the well-known ("super-size me") increase in French-fry servings (high in fat) has resulted in a nearly 60% increase in kcal during that 20-year period. The roughly

Figure 2.7.
Increasing portion sizes of fast foods.

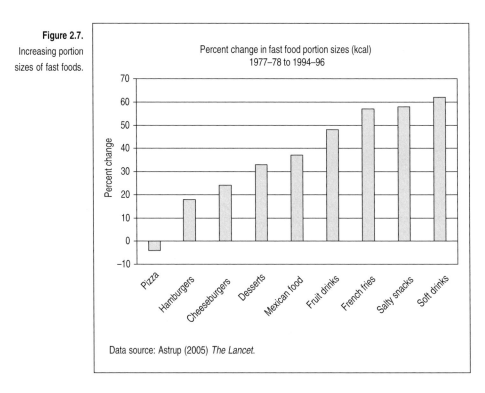

62% increase in kcal in soft drinks due to the larger portion sizes is also noteworthy. Bray, Nielsen, and Popkin (2004) describe the relation between the intake of high fructose corn syrup (the primary sweetener in soft drinks) and the increase in obesity which includes both increased caloric intake and the enhancement of caloric over-consumption (Figure 2.7).

Increased fast food

Pereira and colleagues (2005), using data from the large prospective United States CARDIA population-based study, reported that frequent fast food consumption is associated with weight gain over a 15-year period. These findings, which were adjusted for various potential confounds, are summarized in Figure 2.8. In addition to the significantly greater increases in weight over time, persons who ate meals from fast food restaurants more than twice weekly had over a 100% increase in insulin resistance (which can lead to type II diabetes; see chapter 5) than persons who ate less than one meal at a fast food restaurant per week (Pereira et al., 2005).

A growing body of research has documented the adverse effects of fast food consumption on the dietary quality of overall food intake among children and its likely association to obesity. For example,

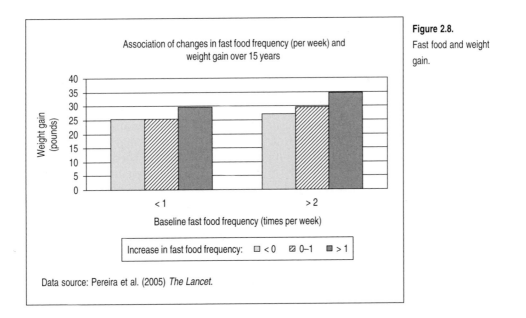

Figure 2.8.
Fast food and weight gain.

Bowman, Gortmaker, Ebbeling, Pereira, & Ludwig (2004), in a study of 6212 children and adolescents aged 4 to 19 years of age in the United States participating in a nationally-representative food intake study in 1994–96 reported several important findings. First, on average, 30.3% of the participants had fast food on any given day. Children who ate fast food on a given day consumed an average of 187 kcal more than children who did not have fast food. Within-subject analyses, a powerful method in which children served as their own control, revealed that children ate more calories and had poorer nutrition on the days they had fast food versus the days they did not have fast food.

Decreased physical activity

In general, physical activity is negatively associated with obesity and with obesity-related morbidity and mortality. Persons who are more physically active are significantly less likely to be obese, to become obese, and to suffer from obesity-related health consequences (Grilo, 1994; Grilo et al., 1993). Physical activity is one of the best (and few) predictors of long-term weight control. Inactivity is a major contri-butor to obesity and recent declines in physical activity are associated with the recent increases in obesity. Figure 2.9 summarizes data from the Schmitz and colleagues (2000) analyses of changes in physical activity and body weight over a ten-year period from the population-based CARDI study. As shown in Figure 2.9, decreases in physical activity are accompanied by increases in body weight in both white and black women.

It is important to emphasize that physical activity encompasses many things, from standing, to walking, to lifestyle activities, to various forms (aerobic, resistance training) and intensities of exercise behaviors. Although many think first of moderate and rigorous forms of exercise, an impressive body of research suggests that regular lifestyle physical activity is a key component of successful long-term weight control (Grilo et al., 1993) and that even moderate fitness results in tremendous health benefits. These issues will be covered further in chapter 6 within the context of interventions for obesity. Even regular walking behaviors are important for understanding weight and obesity. Although walking tends to burn more calories in heavier persons, many – but not all (Browning & Kram, 2005) – studies find that obese persons prefer to walk more slowly.

The important role of everyday physical activity in obesity has been further illuminated by two fascinating studies performed by

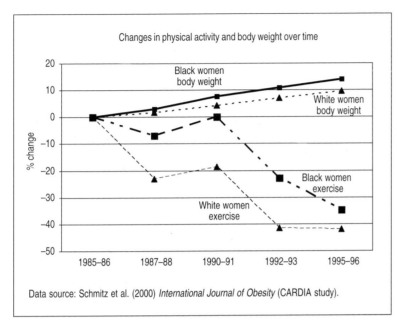

Figure 2.9. Changes in physical activity and body weight over time. Data source: Schmitz et al. (2000) *International Journal of Obesity* (CARDIA study).

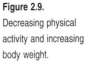

Figure 2.9.
Decreasing physical activity and increasing body weight.

Levine and colleagues (2005). Levine, Eberhardt, and Jensen (1999) described a form of daily physical activity termed NEAT as non-exercise activity thermogenesis. NEAT refers to non-purposeful exercise or physical activity such as sitting, standing, walking, talking, and so on. NEAT was found to increase in order to prevent weight gain in certain persons. Specifically, volunteers who were overfed gained different amounts of weight and the differences in weight gain were associated with differences in NEAT.

Levine and colleagues (2005) expanded on these findings by separating NEAT into two different components: posture (standing, sitting, and lying) versus movement (any walking, etc.). These researchers compared ten lean and ten mildly obese sedentary volunteers using sophisticated measures of energy and movement. These 20 persons had their body postures and movements measured every half-second for 10 days resulting in approximately 25 million data points per person. The results were striking. Obese individuals were seated an average of two hours longer per day than the lean individuals. To determine whether these findings were a cause of consequence of obesity, the researchers performed a second part to the study. The obese persons were put on a diet (and lost 8 kg) and the lean persons were overfed for two months and gained 4 kg). The postural movements or component of NEAT did not change with these diet/weight changes, suggesting that NEAT is a biologically determined physical activity. Levine et al. (2005) reported that the extra NEAT behaviors characteristic of the lean persons accounted for roughly 350 extra kcal burned off per day.

Pima Indians: An example of potent environmental influences

One interesting "natural experiment" to examine the impact of environmental factors such as diet on obesity is to compare groups of persons who move to a different country with a different environment to their biological relatives who remain in their native country. The case of the Pima Indians represents a potent example of the negative effects of environment on a genetically susceptible group of persons. Figure 2.10 summarizes data extracted from a series of studies on the Pima Indians (Fox et al., 1999; Ravussin et al., 1994; Smith et al., 1996). A portion of this tribe from Mexico migrated to

Figure 2.10.
Impact of environment changes on body weight and fat: Observations of the Pima Indians.

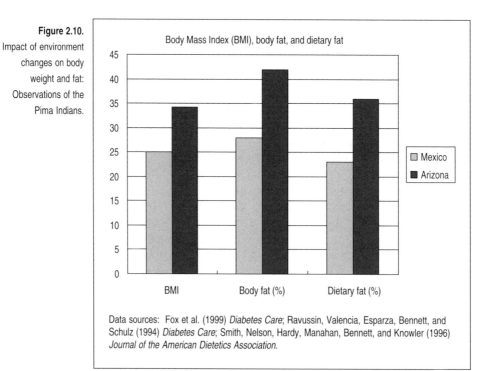

Data sources: Fox et al. (1999) *Diabetes Care*; Ravussin, Valencia, Esparza, Bennett, and Schulz (1994) *Diabetes Care*; Smith, Nelson, Hardy, Manahan, Bennett, and Knowler (1996) *Journal of the American Dietetics Association*.

Arizona and was exposed to a drastically different environmental risk for obesity. As is shown in Figure 2.10, the increases in BMI and in percentage body fat in the Pima Indians in Arizona were commensurate with the percentage increase in dietary fat. Ravussin and colleagues (1994) concluded that despite a potential similar genetic susceptibility to obesity and diabetes, Pima Indians living a "traditional" lifestyle in Mexico (characterized by a lower fat diet and a physically more active lifestyle) may protect against developing obesity and diabetes.

Other factors?

There exist many other factors which may play important roles in the development of obesity, both in individuals as well as at the societal level. For example, several large prospective studies have reported some associations between depression in childhood or adolescence and obesity or weight gain at later points in time. Pine, Cohen, and Brook et al. (1997) found that obesity in adulthood was associated with adolescent depression in females. Richardson and colleagues (2003), in a longitudinal study of a New Zealand birth cohort, found that, among females only, depression in adolescence increased the chances of obesity in young adulthood and also reported a significant dose relationship with number of depressive episodes predicting risk for adult obesity among women. Goodman and Whitaker (2002), in a prospective cohort study of 9374 adolescents in the National Longitudinal Study of Adolescent Health, reported that depressed mood at baseline independently predicted obesity at a follow-up (only one year in contrast to the other longer term studies) later even after controlling for baseline BMI and several important potential confounding variables. Hasler and colleagues (2004), in a prospective community-based cohort study of 591 young adults followed between ages 19 and 40, reported that atypical forms of depression were significantly associated with both increased weight gain and with being obese at follow-up.

In a recent provocative and critical review, Keith and colleagues (in press) emphasized the importance of not neglecting potential factors (other than increased fast food and decreased physical activity) associated with the societal increases in obesity. One example of such a factor is sleep. Research has found that persons who sleep between six and eight hours nightly have lower BMIs than those persons who sleep fewer than five hours or more than nine hours per night (Kripke, Garfinkel, Wingard, Klauber, & Maler, 2002; Patel et al., 2004).

Figure 2.11.

Sleep and body mass

index.

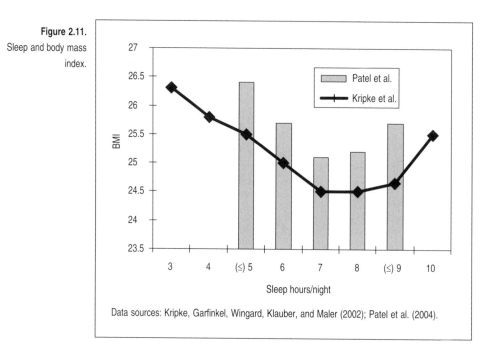

Data sources: Kripke, Garfinkel, Wingard, Klauber, and Maler (2002); Patel et al. (2004).

Findings from two recent large studies on sleep debt are summarized in Figure 2.11 showing that chronic sleep deprivation is associated with increased risk for weight gain. As noted by Keith and colleagues (in press), the average amount of sleep has decreased during the past several decades (Bonnet & Arand, 1995) as the prevalence of obesity has increased.

Keith and colleagues (in press) also presented a number of other potential factors that appear to have changed over time in ways that parallel the increases in obesity. Some of these other factors potentially associated with the societal increase in obesity include, for example, decreased smoking, widespread use of medications that produce weight gain, increasing mothers' ages at childbirth, changes in ethnicity and age distribution, endocrine disrupters, and increasing temperature control (household heating and cooling). These authors emphasized that it is important to study these and a number of other factors potentially associated with the societal increases in obesity. While increased fast food and unhealthy overeating coupled with decreased physical activity are likely important factors, research should not neglect the search and study of other or additional contributors to the obesity epidemic.

Summary

Our society is characterized by pervasive pressures to achieve certain body image ideals (thin and fit) alongside a toxic food environment comprised of plentiful unhealthy high-caloric foods within a lifestyle context of insufficient physical activity and excess eating. Not surprisingly, there is widespread discontent with weight and shape and high rates of ineffective and unhealthy dieting. A small percentage of people develop eating disorders such as anorexia nervosa and bulimia nervosa. These serious eating disorders occur disproportionately in young women in westernized societies. Little is known about the etiology of these eating disorders but emerging research suggests a complex interplay among genetic, biological, temperamental, and psychological factors. A larger percentage of people develop other eating problems such as binge eating, which may be a contributing factor to obesity in some people. In contrast to the low rates of eating disorders, obesity is an extremely common problem that continues to increase in prevalence. Obesity is increasing in prevalence across all age groups, both genders, most ethnic groups, and in many different countries worldwide. Although complex genetic vulnerabilities to develop obesity exist, excess eating and insufficient physical activity are necessary factors.

Understanding, assessing, and treating anorexia nervosa 3

Introduction

Anorexia nervosa (AN) is the least common and the most serious eating disorder. AN is characterized by refusal to maintain a minimal body weight and by extreme weight control methods including severely restricted and controlled eating. These patients have severe disturbances in how they experience and evaluate their bodies. Persons with AN have a remarkable degree of denial about their problem, which unlike the other eating and weight disorders, tends to be "egosyntonic" (i.e., not seen as a problem or something foreign or unwanted by the self). AN results in high rates of serious medical problems and has one of the highest death rates for any psychiatric problem. Despite the seriousness of this problem, limited progress has been achieved either in understanding the nature of this frequently chronic and debilitating disorder or how best to help persons suffering from it (Agras et al., 2004; Fairburn & Harrison, 2003; NICE, 2004; Wilson, 2005). This chapter begins with an overview of the major assessment issues relevant to AN. The major research findings about treatment and management will then be summarized.

Assessment of anorexia nervosa

The challenge

The assessment of anorexia nervosa (AN) is complicated by several factors. The most challenging issue is the denial of the problem. Many persons with AN will deny or refuse to acknowledge that they are underweight or unable to maintain (or work toward) a healthy weight. Since they see and experience themselves as overweight or even "fat," despite the reality of their very thin states, they are very resistant to clear feedback about their weight and medical complications. They frequently have somatic complaints (e.g., feeling cold, fatigue, headaches, and constipation) and insist that they have "special" or different metabolisms. Further, they refuse to acknowledge that many of these somatic complaints are signs and symptoms of serious underlying medical problems that are being caused by the severe starvation and weight loss.

Features and characteristics

AN is characterized by a refusal to maintain a minimal normal body weight, an intense fear of becoming fat, and (in females) amenorrhea. The disturbance in body image is severe, and in addition to the way in which the body is experienced there is an overevaluation of weight and shape in determining self-worth. The restricting AN type achieves the abnormally low weight by severe dieting, fasting, and often by exercising compulsively. The binge/purge AN type achieves the low weight by severe dieting and physical activity, but the remarkable dietary control is intermixed with episodes of binge eating or purging through vomiting or misusing laxatives, enemas, or diuretics. It is not uncommon for patients with AN to alternate between the restricting and the bingeing/purging subtypes at different points in their illness over time. Text Box 3.1 provides a clinical example of a case of anorexia nervosa.

Additional medical and psychological problems

The various extreme behaviors of AN frequently result in a plethora of medical problems. In severe cases, the refusal to eat can lead to death by starvation. Death from severe medical complications that appear in multiple organ systems is not uncommon. These patients are further complicated by high rates of co-occurring additional psychiatric problems and psychological difficulties. The relation between AN and these other problems is challenging to determine. The semi-starvation state makes its difficult to assess these problems and to determine, for example, whether they are primary disorders or direct consequences of the starvation. In addition, suicide is not uncommon and continues to be a major cause of death in this patient group.

General considerations and approach to assessment

Ideally, a comprehensive assessment would involve obtaining information about the nature and specifics of each of the AN behaviors as

TEXT BOX 3.1

Clinical example of anorexia nervosa

A.J. is a 15-year-old-single white female. She was the second of three children in an affluent family living in a suburb of a large city. Her father was chief executive officer of a major company and her mother was a partner in a prestigious law firm. The family frequently entertained and was socially very well connected. The family placed a premium on success. A.J. played two sports and was actively pursued by several prestigious residential private schools. A.J., at her parents' insistence, enrolled at a different elite "prep" school than her older brother. A.J. did well at school but felt somewhat isolated and uncomfortable with her peers despite their similar social status and aspirations. Unlike many of her girlfriends she returned home for the summer lean (given her athletic participation) and *without* having put on any weight. About a week after arriving home, her mother commented to her that she and her father thought it was important that she resume and sustain a vigorous exercise schedule to "keep her edge" for the following school year. A.J. was also enrolled in a specific sports camp and overheard her parents discussing their concerns that she might "get soft."

A.J. worked hard that summer in the sports camp and increased her exercise whenever possible. She became leaner and stronger and received a lot of positive encouragement from her coaches and peers. A.J.'s parents said nothing when she returned home. During the one week after camp and before her return to school, she decided to intensify her diet. During that week, she lost another four pounds primarily by just eating vegetables and lean protein. When she returned to school, her coaches noticed and reinforced her for her condition. Several of her girlfriends also made positive comments.

A.J. became increasingly preoccupied with her weight, her eating, and her exercise. She continued to lose weight. Her roommates did not notice at first but one of her coaches expressed concern that she seemed to be going from being lean to being too thin. This coach initially expressed his concerns in relation to her optimal weight for athletic performance. Soon, this coach became concerned about her health. The coach had several supportive conversations with A.J. but she repeatedly denied she had any problem. She began to dress in layers and lied about her weight during team weigh-ins.

A.J.'s preoccupation with weight and exercise soon became obsessional. She began to spend more and more time alone. She constantly thought about food while managing to eat less and less. There were many days that she ate little more than eggs whites and a few vegetables. On days that she ate other foods she carefully counted (and recounted) calories and made sure to exercise longer to burn off the "extra" calories. She frequently checked and pinched her belly and thighs for any fat despite being underweight. Soon she was checking her body and weighing herself multiple times during the day. She found herself frequently thinking about food but was delighted that she could resist eating, unlike her girlfriends who frequently complained about overeating. When she ate she felt anxious but her calorie counting and exercise behaviors helped her feel in control. She continued to lose weight and soon her athletic performance began to drop off. This led the coach to speak with the parents who expressed concern about her performance but seemed dismissive of the coach's concerns about health. A.J. went home for the holidays about 15 pounds lighter but managed to hide this rather well with her "layered" style of dressing. She said she "liked to feel squishy" in her clothes. Her parents only commented that the coach had concerns about her performance and encouraged her to stay at it. Little changed when she returned to school except for more weight loss. One day, she collapsed in practice and this prompted the school to intervene. The physician called the parents and recommended that they seek specialized care.

continues overleaf

TEXT BOX 3.1

continued

COMMENT

This example reflects a fairly typical clinical presentation characteristic of anorexia nervosa. Anorexia nervosa occurs most frequently in white young females from well-educated and successful families that place a premium on appearance and achievement. Anorexia nervosa occurs most frequently during adolescence and tends to occur after a period of strict dieting, often following some stressful event or negative commentary about body shape or weight. It remains unknown why so many young women diet but so few go on to develop anorexia nervosa. It seems that certain temperaments (obsessional, rigid, perfectionistic types with poor self-esteem) are more likely to develop anorexia nervosa. In these cases, the dieting seems to be rewarding by providing a sense of control or mastery and thus is not experienced as a problem by the person.

well as about each of these associated psychiatric and medical issues. This tends to be a difficult process because the seriousness of the low weight and extreme weight control methods are frequently and steadfastly denied. Three additional general points need to be emphasized.

First, as noted in chapter 1, it is critical not to view the diagnostic requirements for eating disorders too rigidly. This is especially true for AN. The most obvious example is that females with and without amenorrhea (required for the formal diagnosis) do not differ in meaningful ways. Of course the amenorrhea may signal greater endocrine abnormalties and potential for some severe medical consequences, but it is not a great indicator of the psychopathology and clinical challenge that lies ahead. Similarly, a person with these features who is "technically" not quite at the 85% weight criterion still should be regarded as having a severe problem. Moreover, clinical experience suggests that further weight loss, if not prevented, will only serve to intensify (rather than reduce) the intense fear of fatness.

Second, many patients with AN are adolescents. Historically, a previous edition of the DSM (i.e., the third, published in 1980) listed the AN criteria in the section on disorders of children and adolescents. Since less research has focused on adolescents than adults, it is even more difficult to arrive at firm conclusions regarding diagnostic, assessment, or treatment issues for this age group (Eating Disorders Commission, 2005). Some of the criteria for AN are arguably more ambiguous in adolescents. For example, determining ideal weight, ideal growth and maturation, and when weight loss is excessive, is more uncertain in adolescents than in adults. A separate issue concerns the general challenge in establishing rapport and eliciting accurate information from young people during this developmental era. In addition to high self-consciousness which may influence disclosure, there is the added complexity of the normal turbulence of adolescence and the well-known difficulties in accurate reporting about time and events. Since many of these problems are kept secret from parents, parental corroboration is difficult at best.

Third, assessment is an ongoing dynamic process. For most psychiatric problems, ongoing assessment is an integral part of the most effective interventions. Ongoing assessment allows for tracking of progress as well as guiding subsequent steps in the treatment process. In AN, this approach is critically important for these reasons as well as for factors specific to the illness. The egosyntonic nature of AN dictates the need for constant monitoring of all of aspects of the AN including frequency and intensity of behaviors and cognitions, weight changes, and medical status. The well-known alternations or symptom fluctuations (Tozzi et al., 2005) dictate ongoing assessments. Such ongoing assessments reveal targets for additional interventions. Such assessments are important for determining medical risk. For example, as will be described below, the development of purging in a low-weight restricting AN patient increases the risk for serious cardiac complications.

Assessment instruments and anorexia nervosa

Many of the issues reviewed above are assessed via traditional clinical interviewing. An important advance in the psychiatry field has been the development of semi-structured interviews to facilitate comprehensive evaluations of specific problems. These methods offer a number of important strengths, including the systematic exploration of problems which decreases the chances of missing important features. From a research perspective these standardized methods allow for clear communication and comparison across research studies. The interested reader is referred to the Mitchell and Peterson (2005) volume on assessment methods for eating disorders and Grilo, Lozano, and Elder's (2005) review of structured interviewing methods.

There are several structured interviews developed specifically for assessing the features of eating disorders. Currently, the best established of these interviews is the Eating Disorder Examination

(EDE; Fairburn & Cooper, 1993), a standardized semi-structured investigator-based approach. The EDE assesses the features of eating disorders and allows for determining the specific ED diagnoses. The EDE has shown good diagnostic properties and is widely considered a rigorous measure for assessing diverse eating disorder psycho-pathology (Grilo et al., 2001a, 2001b; Grilo, Lozano, & Elder, 2005; Grilo et al., 2004a). The EDE has been adapted for use with children and adolescents (ChEDE; Bryant-Waugh, Cooper, Taylor, & Lask, 1996) but the utility of this version is not yet known. Neither version of the EDE has been used much in treatment research for AN, unlike the extensive use of the EDE in treatment studies with BN and BED.

In terms of determining diagnoses of eating disorders as well as the presence of other psychiatric diagnoses, there are two primary instruments. For adults, the *Structured Clinical Interview for DSM-IV* (SCID-I/P; First, Spitzer, Gibbon, & Williams, 1996) is the most widely used and established diagnostic interview for DSM-IV axis I psychiatric disorders. For adolescents, the *Schedule for Affective Disorder and Schizophrenia for School-Age Children* (K-SADS; Orvaschel & Puig-Antich, 1987) is the clear standard.

It is frequently not possible to use these structured interviews for a variety of reasons, including the need for skilled clinical interviewers, time burden, and costs. There exist a large number of self-report questionnaires for assessing different aspects and features of eating disorders (Mitchell & Peterson, 2005). There is considerable vari-ability in these questionnaires and pros and cons to using them (Grilo, Masheb, & Wilson, 2001b). Two frequently used self-report questionnaires with research backing for their general utility are the *Eating Disorder Examination-Questionnaire Version* (EDE-Q; Fairburn & Beglin, 1994) and the *Questionnaire for Eating and Weight Patterns – Revised* (QEWP-R; Yanovski, 1993). These two self-report question-naires require relatively little time for persons to complete and can provide a wealth of information to clinicians and researchers. The ease with which these assessments can be given and scored make them valuable tools to assess changes in symptom severity over the course of treatment. The few research studies conducted to date comparing self-report to structured interviews have suggested that self-report methods are less useful for younger groups than for older persons, yet they can provide some useful information (Binford, LeGrange, & Jellar, 2004; Passi, Bryson, & Lock, 2003). Many times, the self-report instruments are used to identify potential problems and if it seems that problems are likely they are then followed up using interviews.

Medical assessment of anorexia nervosa

Medical assessment of AN is a complex but critically important process. Some persons with AN show no obvious signs or evidence of medical problems. The prolonged starvation, however, affects most organ systems and a wide array of serious medical problems are frequently present (Schoken, Holloway, & Powers, 1989; Sharp & Freeman, 1993). The remarkable struggles that can ensue around eating and weight can sometimes overshadow the need for active vigilance and management of the serious medical complications that very frequently develop in these patients. In general, a combination of lower weight and purging behaviors is associated with greater medical risk including death. Table 3.1 summarizes the major body systems that are influenced by AN as well as the most common medical problems seen in these patients.

The severe restriction of caloric (and fluid) intake in the restricting type AN patients and the added purging behaviors in the binge/ purge types stress many of the body's homeostatic processes and can impact on nearly every major organ system. Disrupted fluid homeostasis and electrolyte abnormalities are common and are extremely dangerous and life threatening. Hypokalemia, the most frequent electrolyte abnormality, which occurs due to potassium loss especially in frequent purgers, can result in cardiac arrhythmias. This is one of the major causes of death in AN patients. Hypokalemia can also lead to nephropathy and renal failure. Severe restriction, especially when fluid intake is decreased, frequently results in a hypovolemic state which triggers the body's efforts to achieve homeostasis by conserving fluids. This is seen most frequently in those patients who abuse laxatives and diuretics. This requires careful monitoring when helping these patients "withdraw" from their use of these substances. Constipation is nearly universal in such cases and patients require persistent support to prevent them from returning to laxatives.

A plethora of cardiac abnormalities are common in AN patients. These range from the serious arrhythmias in patients with electrolyte imbalances noted above to forms of sinus arrhythmia and sinus bradycardia that are common but less serious. AN patients have a multitude of gastrointestinal problems, endocrine abnormalities (many reflecting the hypothalamic-pituitary axes), and dermatological problems. Some of the dermatological problems provide clues to clinicians and family members who suspect AN. Hair loss is common along with a growth of facial hair ("lanugo"). Since this occurs in

TABLE 3.1

Common physical and medical issues associated with anorexia nervosa

Renal and electrolyte problems
- Electrolyte abnormalities and disrupted fluid homeostasis can occur in severely restricting patients. Low weight AN binge/purge subtype patients who self-induce vomiting and abuse laxatives are at significant risk. Most common and serious electrolyte abnormality is hypokalemia (potassium loss), which can result in cardiac arrhythymias.
- Hypovolemic state can occur with severe restriction especially when fluid intake is decreased. This triggers the body's efforts to achieve homeostasis by conserving fluids.

Cardiovascular system
- Cardiac events are one of major causes of death.
- Cardiac abnormalities are common in very low weight highly restrictive patients.
- AN binge/purge subtypes who purge frequently are also at risk for electrolyte abnormalties such as hypokalemia which can trigger cardiac arrhythmias. These instances are considered the most dangerous and potentially fatal.
- Hypotension common due to dehydration from severe restriction.

Gastrointestinal system
- Purging subtypes have higher risk of GI problems.

Endocrine system
- Endocrine abnormalties are frequent and extensive in AN.
- Some abnormalties reflect hypothalamic-pituitary (HP) axes.

Metabolic problems
- Osteopenia (decreased or low bone density) is a frequent problem.

Dermatological system
- Hair loss (from the head) and "lanugo" hair (fine facial hair) occur in 30% to 50% cases.
- Excessively dry skin, orange discoloration of skin, and brittle nails are common.

Reproductive system
- Obstetrical complications are common.

roughly 30% to 50% cases, being alert to it can help to identify many individuals. Other common dermatological signs include dry skin, orange discoloration of skin, and brittle nails. This is noteworthy because these are common complaints in patients even when they deny having a problem with eating or weight.

One of the most serious medical complications in AN is osteopenia, which refers to decreased or low bone density. This is likely a consequence of amenorrhea and low estrogen levels as well as malnutrition (Grinspoon et al., 2000). It is noteworthy that such decreases in bone density can occur quickly and relatively soon after the AN develops (Bachrach, Guido, Katzman, Litt, & Marcus, 1990). It is not unusual to find bone densities in these young women as low as typically seen in cases of post-menopausal osteoporosis. Increased fracture risk is therefore present. Osteopenia frequently persists after recovery from AN and does not seem reversible in some patients (Bachrach, Katzman, Litt, Guido, & Marcus, 1991). Effective interventions for this serious problem have yet to be determined (Grinspoon, Thomas, Miller, Herzog, & Klibanski, 2002).

AN has serious complications for reproductive function and child bearing. If these patients eventually become pregnant, numerous psychological and medical challenges may continue to exist. Drastic changes in weight and body shape with the pregnancy can be frightening to some "recovered" AN patients. Relapse is not uncommon in these patients if they become pregnant. Kouba, Hallstrom, Lindholm, and Hirschberg (2005) reported that 22% of a sample of 49 women previously diagnosed with eating disorders relapsed during their pregnancy and Franko and colleagues (2001) reported elevated rates of post-partum depression. Higher rates of miscarriage, various obstetric complications are common, and babies are at risk for lower weight (Kouba et al., 2005). The interested reader is referred to Franko and Spurrell (2000) for useful guidelines to help detect and to collaboratively manage eating disorders during pregnancy.

Lastly, a detailed list of laboratory tests that can be used to assess common physical complications of anorexia nervosa across the various organ systems can be found in the *Revised Practice Guidelines for the Treatment of Patients With Eating Disorders* (American Psychiatric Association, 2004).

Psychological assessment of anorexia nervosa

Persons with AN have high lifetime rates of other psychiatric problems and it is not unusual for these persons to suffer from several additional disorders. The pattern of the difficulties is diverse and complex. A general observation is that community samples of AN have fewer co-occurring problems than outpatient samples which, in turn, have fewer co-occurring problems than inpatient samples. Higher rates of co-occurring problems in the clinical groups may reflect greater severity in the AN or greater psychiatric problems in general that lead to increased treatment seeking.

There is considerable variability in the sequence of when these persons develop other psychiatric problems. Sometimes other psychiatric problems occur before, sometimes at about the same time, and frequently after the AN develops. It is often difficult to determine whether these additional problems reflect secondary effects of the starvation (Keys et al., 1950) or the co-existence of those psychiatric disorders.

These findings and issues make it important to assess what other major psychiatric or psychological problems may be present in persons with AN. Although the significance of co-occurring psychiatric problems for understanding the underlying nature of AN is uncertain, it is important to determine the presence of other problems. This is essential for good clinical management and for determining treatments.

Many studies with treatment-seeking clinical groups report that roughly 80% of patients with AN have at least one additional psychiatric disorder over their lifetime (Halmi, Eckert, Marchi, Sampugnaro, Apple, & Cohen, 1991). Certain psychiatric problems are especially common in patients with AN. The most common additional specific disorder is major depressive disorder, which is generally experienced by 50% to 70% of patients (Herzog, Keller, Sacks, Yeh, & Lavori, 1992; Halmi et al., 1991). Anxiety disorders as a group are extremely common in AN patients, with reports generally finding about 50% to 65% lifetime rates; social phobia and obsessive-compulsive disorder are the most commonly seen specific forms of anxiety (Halmi et al., 1991; Herzog et al., 1992; see review by Herzog, Nussbaum, & Marmor, 1996). Substance use disorders are found in roughly 10% to 20% of AN patients (Herzog et al., 1992; Stock, Goldberg, Corbett, & Katzman, 2002). This rate is higher than estimates for young females without eating disorders in the general population but is slightly lower than estimates for women with bulimia nervosa (Bulik, Sullivan, McKee, Weltzin, & Kaye, 1994). Consistent with this finding, studies have reported that the binge/purge type of AN is more likely than the restricting type of AN to have a substance use disorder (Herzog et al., 1992; Stock et al., 2002). Noteworthy is that alcohol use disorders were predictive of mortality in AN (Keel et al., 2003). Personality disorders, most notably the cluster C "anxious and fearful" disorders (avoidant, dependant, and obsessive-compulsive personality disorders) are common in AN.

Research has observed variability in the sequence of when AN patients develop these various other psychiatric problems (Anderluh et al., 2003; Braun, Sunday, & Halmi, 1994; Bulik, Sullivan, Fear, &

Joyce, 1997a). The onset of major depressive disorder seems variable between individuals and has been reported to occur before, during, and after episodes of AN. There are several reports that anxiety disorders more frequently precede AN and that substance use disorders most frequently follow AN.

Several studies have attempted to compare the nature and extent of additional general psychopathology in younger versus older groups of patients with AN. Halmi, Casper, Eckert, Goldberg, and Davis (1979) reported that AN patients with a younger onset tended to have higher frequencies of some of the eating disorder behaviors but general psychological features and levels of psychopathology were similar for younger versus later onset cases. More recently, Cooper, Watkins, Bryant-Waugh, and Lask (2002) reported that both eating disorder psychopathology and general psychopathology were essentially the same in early versus late onset AN patients. These findings suggest that adolescents and adults with AN are generally similar in their clinical presentations.

Overview of treatments for anorexia nervosa

There has been very little treatment research, particularly controlled studies, for AN. The paucity of research is due to several factors. First, this is a relatively rare disorder and most patients deny the existence of a problem and go to considerable lengths to disguise their underweight state. Even when persons with AN are identified and strongly encouraged to seek treatment and are supported during the process, they are often highly resistant. Thus, it is not surprising that research centers worldwide have tremendous difficulty recruiting patients for treatment studies (Agras et al., 2004). Moreover, in this patient group that often requires long-term management, discontinuation or dropout from treatment ("attrition") is high and is a major challenge to caregivers and therapists (Strober, 2004). For example, a recent treatment study conducted at three specialized university-based centers found that 46% of patients with AN dropped out from treatment (Halmi et al., 2005). These issues represent considerable challenges to researchers that must be overcome in order to advance our understanding of how best to help these patients.

With the above context in mind, it becomes more understandable why there are so few controlled studies for AN (Fairburn & Harrison,

2003; NICE, 2004). Moreover, most treatment studies for AN suffer from serious methodological limitations. Common problems include absence of control conditions, poorly defined treatments, small sample sizes, high attrition rates, assessments that are narrow or of uncertain quality, and modest follow-up rates.

Overall, even with intensive treatment over time, most studies find that only approximately 50% of anorexia nervosa patients recover and that 20% show a chronic and disabling course (Beumont, Russell, & Touyz, 1993; Steinhausen, 2002; Zipfel et al., 2000). Ben-Tovim, Walker, Gilchrist, Freeman, Kalucy, & Esterman (2001), in a prospective five-year study of a representative sample of ED patients treated in South Australia, found that the recovery rate for AN (56%) was lower than observed for either BN (74%) or EDNOS (78%). This study, which further explored the effects of different treatments including specialist programs, albeit in a naturalistic non-controlled fashion, found that different treatments seemed to exert little influence on the outcomes. Mortality from anorexia nervosa continues to be high and is estimated at 5.6% per decade (Sullivan, 1995). A recently completed 20-year study of a large cohort of patients with AN in Canada confirmed the high mortality rate for this patient group (Birmingham, Su, Hlynsky, Goldner, & Gao, 2005). With this context in mind, an overview of current thinking about how to treat and manage patients with AN follows. This will include a brief review of the small body of treatment research.

Weight restoration and nutritional rehabilitation

Fairburn & Harrison (2003) note that the current expert opinion regarding the treatment of AN includes a few basic concepts. The basic concepts and empirical guidance have changed little from previous expert summaries (Beumont et al., 1993). The first major task is to help persons with AN realize that they have a serious problem and to motivate them to enter into and stay engaged in treatment. The second major task is weight restoration. Because the starvation and weight loss can be life threatening, initial treatment efforts need to focus primarily on weight regain and the re-establishment of eating ("re-feeding"). In many cases, weight regain results in moderate improvement in the patient's overall mental status.

In contrast to the other eating disorders, which are most frequently and adequately treated on an outpatient basis, the treatment of AN frequently requires more intensive approaches such as partial or day hospitalizations in which patients spend much of the day in treatment activities (Kaplan & Olmsted, 1997) or inpatient hospitalizations (Andersen, Bowers, & Evans, 1997). Clear indications for inpatient hospitalization include suicidality, immediate medical danger requiring stabilization, insufficient benefit or worsening of condition despite outpatient treatment, severe familial and interpersonal turmoil in the home, or associated deterioration in mental status and functioning. These intensive treatment options are also frequently chosen when clinical impression suggests that they are needed to prevent further weight loss (i.e., outpatient treatment appears insufficient) or to stabilize the low weight and any associated medical complications. Many clinicians believe that such intensive day or inpatient services are needed to aggressively initiate the challenging process of weight restoration and nutritional rehabilitation.

Level or intensity of treatment

The question of outpatient versus inpatient treatment (except for clear indications because of dangerously low weight, medical complications, clear outpatient failure, or suicidality) for AN remains uncertain. No randomized controlled studies have addressed this question. Reviews of the outcomes produced by programs of different intensities reveal mixed findings at least in terms of their longer term outcomes (Ben-Tovim et al., 2001; Gowers et al., 2000; Meads, Gold, & Burls, 2001; Zipfel et al., 2002). Gowers and colleagues (2000), for example, found for a series of adolescents with AN, the 21 cases that received inpatient care had a significantly worse longer term outcome (two to seven years later at follow-up) than 51 cases that were not admitted to the hospital but were treated as outpatients. This important study highlights the need for further study of the merits of inpatient treatment for AN. The authors concluded in noting that the potential negative consequences of such intensive treatments have been neglected by researchers.

The study by Gowers and colleagues (2000) goes against prevailing clinical lore that more intensive treatments are likely to somehow be better. It is important to note, however, that in the absence of randomized assignment as a control, the findings must be viewed extremely cautiously. Quite simply, patients with greater severity and who are treatment refractory are more likely to be admitted and to receive more treatment. Thus, it is difficult to determine whether it was the greater severity in the inpatients or the intensive treatment that accounted for the poorer outcomes. For example, Ben-Tovim and colleagues (2001) reported that greater severity or intensity of AN symptoms predicted worse five-year outcomes, whereas different treatments made little difference. These questions are important to pursue in research. Clinically, this raises a different issue. In the absence of empirical support for certain interventions, it can be hypothesized that inpatient treatment might simply provide more time with ineffective treatments or allow for a "grab-bag" of treatments and activities of uncertain therapeutic value to be given. These issues require study to resolve.

Dietary regimens

There is consensus that re-establishment of eating and weight restoration are primary treatment tasks. It is critical to prevent any further weight loss in these low weight patients. The lower the weight, the greater the medical risk and in the majority of cases as weight drops the more obsessional, resistant, and fearful the patient becomes. Re-establishment of eating and weight gain must occur before any meaningful psychotherapy is possible. A consistent finding is that greater weight regain and higher weight at discharge from hospitalization predicted better eventual outcome (Baran, Weltzin, & Kaye, 1995; Castro, Gila, Puig, Rodriguez, & Toto, 2004; Howard, Evans, Quintero-Howard, Bowers, & Anderson, 1999). There is no consensus, however, about how to best perform the re-feeding and which behavioral approaches are most advantageous.

Behavioral approaches based on learning theories (e.g., operant conditioning) date back to the 1950s but research has not consistently supported a particular approach. Increasing weight quickly and as much as possible during treatment is critical, and operant conditioning forms of behavior therapy facilitate faster weight gain (Agras, Barlow, Chapin, Abel, & Leitenberg, 1974; Agras & Kraemer, 1983). Broadly speaking, these approaches involve making weight gain a requirement for obtaining reinforcers (i.e., material reinforcers such as music or television and social reinforcers such as more privileges and activities on the psychiatric units and receiving social visitors, etc.) and decreasing opportunities to exercise or purge food. Studies that have compared relatively lenient versus strict operant conditioning forms of behavior therapy to re-feeding patients with anorexia nervosa have reported few differences (Touyz, Beumont, Glaun, Phillips, & Crowie,

1984). This has led some experts (Beumont, Russell, & Touyz, 1993) to advocate for a more lenient and flexible approach since it is more practical in many treatment settings. For detailed descriptions of such behavioral programs and how they can be carried out in hospital programs see Touyz, Beumont, and Dunn (1987).

Nasogastric tube feeding

Although tube feeding is sometimes used in severe cases and is frequently the topic of heated debate, relatively little research has examined its effectiveness. Clinically, tube feeding seems to be a viable approach to help those patients who are incapable of re-establishing oral eating. Tube feeding seems useful for producing rapid initial weight during the early stages of treatment with severely low weight patients who experience intense physical and emotional distress when they eat a "large" volume of food necessary for weight gain. Robb and colleagues (2002), based on a nonrandomized retrospective review of 100 hospitalized adolescent girls with anorexia nervosa, found that the 52 girls who received (voluntary) nocturnal tube feeding gained more than twice as much weight than the 48 girls who did not receive tube feeding. The advantage of the tube feeding was observed even after controlling for the fact that the patients who received tube feeding had more previous hospitalizations and thus were potentially more severe cases. A more recent larger (non-randomized retrospective chart review) study with 381 female inpatients with anorexia nervosa also reported that patients who received tube feeding gained significantly more weight per week than those who were re-fed with standard oral approaches (Zuercher, Cumella, Woods, Eberly, & Carr, 2003). Patients who were tube fed did not differ from those only orally fed in their psychological changes, treatment satisfaction, or medical complications. Zuercher and colleagues (2003) concluded that tube feeding represents a viable and safe method for enhancing outcomes for anorexia nervosa when used in intensive inpatient facilities that can manage medical risks associated with the tube feeding and rapid weight gain.

Psychological treatments

In addition to the necessary weight restoration and nutritional rehabilitation, treatment must address the core psychopathology of

AN which involves the remarkable disturbances in the body image and evaluation. Treatments must address both the intense fear of gaining weight coupled with a relentless pursuit of thinness and the preoccupation with and overevaluation of shape and weight. These core cognitive features and their relation to both ongoing eating behaviors and to psychosocial, interpersonal, and familial functioning require modification. How best to do this remains uncertain. Although many associated psychological symptoms (e.g., depressed, anxious, irritable mood; preoccupation with food; decreased concentration, energy, and interest; social isolation) characteristic of semi-starvation (Keys et al., 1950) show some improvement with weight restoration, the core body image disturbances and links to psychosocial deficits typically remain entrenched and must be addressed (Windauer, Lennerts, Talbot, Touyz, & Beumont, 1993). There are remarkably few controlled studies with any clearly defined interventions for AN that address these core cognitive features and associated psychosocial deficits (NICE, 2004) and this is especially true for adults with AN (Hay, Bacaltchuk, & Stefano, 2003).

Family therapy: The Maudsley Method

The one notable exception is the empirical support for a highly specific form of family therapy for adolescents developed at the Maudsley Hospital in London by Gerald Russell and his colleagues (Russell et al., 1987). This highly specific behavioral family therapy (frequently referred to as the "Maudsley Method") has been tested in a complex series of studies and has documented effectiveness (Russell et al., 1987) including sustained and superior benefits five years later (Eisler, Dare, Russell, Szmukler, le Grange, & Dodge, 1997). In the series of studies, the family therapy was delivered, on average, in 20 sessions over 12 months. These investigators noted, however, that due to clinical and pragmatic realities the actual intensity (number of sessions) and duration (length of time) varied considerably across families, although these factors seemed unrelated to treatment outcomes. Lock and colleagues (2005) recently reported their findings from a controlled study designed specifically to test the optimal length of the Maudsley family therapy method. Lock et al. (2005) found, in a study of 84 adolescents with AN, that a short-term therapy (ten sessions over six months) was as effective as a longer term therapy (20 sessions over 12 months) for those patients who had AN for a shorter duration. However, for adolescents with longer durations of AN, with more severe obsessive thinking, and with non-intact families, the longer treatment approach seemed more beneficial.

This specific form of family therapy has been described in a published treatment manual (Lock & Le Grange, 2001; Lock et al., 2001), although the treatment continues to undergo testing and further refinement (Lock et al., 2005). It is important to emphasize that there are many general and different approaches to family therapy. It is also important to note that it remains unknown whether other treatment or research centers can replicate the outcomes reported by its developers. The interested reader is referred to Dare and Eisler (1997) for a detailed presentation of the different theoretical models that guide diverse family interventions and a comparison of the Maudsley Method to other approaches to family therapy with a focus on how the clinical conceptualizations guide the clinician when interacting with the families. Text Box 3.2 provides a brief overview of the Maudsley Method of family therapy for AN.

These research findings support this specific approach and cannot generalize to more traditional family interventions. This approach has received further general support in additional treatment studies that have tested different methods of providing the treatment (e.g., conjoint versus separate family sessions; Eisler et al., 2000) and against different forms of psychotherapy (Robin, Siegel, Koepke, Moye, & Tice, 1994; Robin, Siegel, Moye, Gilroy, Dennis, & Sikand, 1999; Russell et al., 1987). For example, Russell et al. (1987) in a one-year treatment study with 57 patients with AN found that Maudsley Method family therapy was more effective than individual supportive psychotherapy in younger patients (before age 19) whose illness was not chronic. In contrast, a smaller study with 25 hospitalized adolescent girls with AN found no differences between a more "generic" family therapy versus a family group psychoeducation control (Geist, Heinmaa, Stephens, Davis, & Katzman, 2000). Although Geist and colleagues (2000) concluded that the less expensive method (group psychoeducation) was equally an effective method for providing treatment, the fact that neither of these generic family interventions resulted in any changes in psychological or eating disorder features argues against such recommendations. Given the specific support documented for the Maudsley Method, it is encouraging that there is ongoing research (Eating Disorders Commission, 2005) testing additional modifications and variations of this approach to helping families with a family member suffering from AN. It is especially important for clinical researchers other than its developers to test this treatment approach in additional settings.

TEXT BOX 3.2

Maudsley Model of Family Therapy for anorexia nervosa

The Maudsley Model (and "Method") for Family Therapy refers to the approach developed at the Maudsley Hospial in London. The theoretical model and treatment methods date back to the seminal work of Drs. Russell, Szmukler, Dare, and Eisler (1987). The Maudsley Model has continued to evolve further in collaboration with their colleagues (Eisler, Dare, Hodes, Russell, Dodge, & Le Grange, 2000; Lock, Agras, Bryson, & Kraemer, 2005). A published manual is available (Lock, Grange, Agras, & Dare, 2001) for the interested reader. A brief overview of the model follows. Readers interested in a more detailed description of the approach and its distinctiveness from other family therapies can review Dare and Eisler (1997).

The Maudsley Model proposes that AN is a complex illness that results from "multifactorial" etiological influences (Dare & Eisler, 1997). It holds that an "interactional systems" model is the best way to understand the multiple factors that come together to create or cause AN ("etiology") and serve to perpetuate ("maintain") the problem. Genetic (and biological) and social (and cultural) factors affect both the family and the individual with AN. There is a lifecycle (typical developmental process) that is created by interacting with the genetic and social context. The family and the individual influence each other throughout the lifecycle and this occurs within the biological-social context. The AN symptoms (e.g., starvation) arise from the complex not yet understood etiological factors. AN symptoms influence *both* the family and the individual and are influenced by *both* the family and the individual. As long as the symptoms persist, they influence the course of the lifecycle.

The Maudsley Method or approach to family therapy is guided by the above interactional system model. This family therapy method is a structured, active and collaborative approach. The therapy focuses on the behavioral and cognitive symptoms of AN. The adolescent with AN is viewed as incapable of maintaining an appropriate weight for age and gender and is at risk for becoming incapacitated because of the symptoms and their dangerous consequences. The family therapist provides structure, consistency, and support throughout the course of treatment. The family therapist provides information about AN including what is known about it and possible associated complications and what to expect in the treatment. Typically, the family therapist meets briefly individually with the adolescent AN patient and then holds a longer meeting with the entire family. It is not unusual, especially during the early phases of therapy, for brief focused phone meetings to be held in between meetings to address problems.

The first phase of therapy is re-feeding to produce weight gain. The family therapist enlists and attempts to unite the parents and family in developing and agreeing to a consistent approach to eating and re-feeding. This process is facilitated by reviewing and emphasizing with the family's struggles and frustrations in trying to help the child or adolescent. It is frequently necessary to address and dispel parental concerns that they "caused" the eating disorder and it is sometimes necessary to address frustrations that the child or adolescent can simply begin to eat normally if they so desired. The therapist provides support and feedback but it is the parents who develop and carry out the re-feeding. Whenever possible, the therapist enlists siblings to support the AN person.

The second phase of therapy begins once steady weight gain occurs and there is both relief and confidence that the family has achieved some progress and re-established some control over the AN. The therapy continues to focus on the behavioral and cognitive features of the AN but the focus broadens and begins to consider other challenges and issues. Frequently,

continues

stressors include social situations (e.g., eating at school, attending parties, etc.) and seemingly basic activities (exercise, sports participation, etc.) that can be major pitfalls if not handled carefully.

The third phase begins after a stable appropriate weight is achieved and there are minimal struggles with eating. This phase focuses on other concerns that have been put on hold because of the prioritized focus on re-feeding and weight stabilization. There is often improvement in other areas once the starvation is eliminated and a reasonable weight is established. The family and individual now have more resources to be able to address other issues that face all the family members. Typical developmental issues include more independence or autonomy for adolescents, adjusting family boundaries as appropriate, and revisiting parental roles as the adolescent re-establishes healthier behaviors.

More recently, two randomized controlled trials have tested specific outpatient treatments for adults with AN (Dare, Eisler, Russell, Treasure, & Dodge, 2001; McIntosh et al., 2005). Dare and colleagues (2001) reported that family therapy and a psychoanalytic psychotherapy were superior to a control condition. McIntosh and colleagues (2005) reported that a nonspecific supportive clinical management method was superior to interpersonal psychotherapy, while cognitive behavioral therapy (CBT) was intermediate to the other two treatments. Interestingly, Russell and colleagues (1987) in the earlier study noted above that reported the superiority of the Maudsley Method for younger cases of AN noted a tentative finding that individual supportive therapy was more beneficial for older patients.

Pharmacotherapy

Various medications (antipsychotics, antidepressants, anxiolytics, appetite-enhancing agents, prokinetic agents) have been tested for anorexia nervosa without much success. Although the literature is peppered with open-label case reports regarding potential promise of medications for promoting weight gain, the few controlled studies have consistently failed to support their usefulness (Attia, Haiman, Walsh, & Flater, 1998; Biederman et al., 1985; Halmi, Eckert, LaDu, & Cohen, 1986; Vandereycken, 1984). Medications have not been found to promote weight gain in this patient group. Medications have also not been found to improve eating disorder psychopathology in AN patients nor to improve associated general psychopathology. Thus, at present, there is no established role for pharmacotherapy for the treatment of AN.

Although it is commonplace in clinical practice to use concurrent pharmacotherapy (as part of multimodal treatments), it remains uncertain whether any additive effect occurs. Attia and colleagues (1998) at Columbia University conducted a randomized, placebo-controlled, double-blind study to test whether seven weeks of fluoxetine significantly enhanced a structured intensive inpatient program for AN. This small controlled study with 31 AN patients reported no significant findings on any measure between patients receiving fluoxetine and patients receiving placebo. No differences were observed in weight changes, various measures of eating disorder psychopathology, or general psychopathology (e.g., depression, obsessive-compulsiveness). The authors concluded that pharmacotherapy with fluoxetine does not add any significant benefit to traditional inpatient treatment for AN.

Two controlled studies (using randomized double-blind placebo control) recently tested a different potential role for pharmacotherapy in the management of AN – i.e., does it help prevent relapse in treated and weight restored patients (Kaye et al. 2001; Walsh et al. 2005). In the first study, Kaye and colleagues (2001) tested whether pharmacotherapy with fluoxetine enhances outcomes or prevents relapse in AN patients after intensive inpatient treatment and successful weight restoration. Thirty-five patients with AN who achieved weight restoration with intensive inpatient treatment were randomized to receive either fluoxetine or placebo treatments (in addition to uncontrolled outpatient therapy) for a year following hospital discharge. Sixty-three percent of patients receiving fluoxetine versus 16% receiving placebo completed the 12-month study. Patients receiving fluoxetine who completed the 12-month treatment had lower relapse rates than the other patients. This preliminary study suggested the potential usefulness of adding fluoxetine to outpatient therapy for preventing relapse in weight restored AN.

A more recent larger controlled study conducted at two specialist eating disorder centers (Columbia University and the University of Toronto) also tested whether fluoxetine reduced the rate of relapse in patients with AN following inpatient treatment and weight restoration (Walsh et al., 2005). Ninety-three AN patients who had completed inpatient treatments and had achieved at least 90% of ideal weight were randomized to receive, in double-blind fashion, either fluoxetine or placebo. The medication treatments were provided in addition to individual cognitive behavioral therapy (which was provided by expert clinicians) for one year following hospitalization. Exhaustive analyses failed to reveal any differences in time to relapse or course of the AN in patients who received fluoxetine versus placebo. This carefully executed study indicates that fluoxetine does not provide any added benefits to AN patients receiving CBT even after weight restoration.

Involuntary treatment

It is not uncommon for patients with severe or life-threatening anorexia nervosa to refuse treatment or hospitalization. This raises a complex and highly controversial issue of involuntary treatment and commitment. There is controversy about involuntary treatment in both the law and in mental health. In the area of eating disorders, it is even more complex because most patients are not globally incompetent although some may have impaired judgment and are no longer able to care for themselves (Appelbaum & Rumpf, 1998; Carney, Tait, Saunders, Touyz, & Beumont, 2003; Russell, 2001). It is worth noting that an involuntary or compulsory hospitalization for anorexia nervosa does not necessarily mean nor require compulsory or forced treatment such as forced tube feeding, as opposed to voluntary tube feeding reviewed above (see Russell, 2001). The interested reader is referred to an outstanding multidisciplinary overview by Carney and colleagues (2003) of this issue that cuts across law, psychiatry, psychology, and the social sciences.

Relatively little empirical research has examined the effects of involuntary treatment on patients with anorexia nervosa. Ramsay, Ward, Treasure, and Russell (1999) compared 81 patients with AN who received compulsory treatment to 81 patients with AN who received treatment voluntarily. The patients receiving compulsory treatment gained the same amount of weight as did the voluntary patients although it required slightly longer time to do so. This suggests the short-term utility of involuntary treatment. A follow-up of these patients performed 5.7 years later revealed that more deaths occurred among the compulsory patients (13%) than voluntary patients (2%). The authors noted, however, that the higher term mortality rate among the patients who had received compulsory treatment was likely due to their more severe or refractory conditions (they had more severe histories of abuse, self-harm, and more prior hospitalizations). More recent study examined this issue in a consecutive series of 397 patients with AN admitted to an inpatient program over a seven-year period (Watson, Bowers, & Anderson,

2000). The first finding was that involuntary legal commitment was not uncommon; 16.6% of the patients received compulsory treatment. The compulsory patients were lower in weight at admission, had significantly longer durations of AN, and more previous hospitalizations than the voluntary patients. The compulsory and voluntary patients did not differ in the amount of weight gain (2.6 pounds per week versus 2.2 pounds per week) during the hospitalization. Watson and colleagues (2000) concluded that despite the involuntary initiation of treatment, the legally committed patients with AN derived as much benefit from treatment as the voluntary patients. Thus, even severely ill patients with AN who do not see the need for treatment and are hospitalized by legal commitment do derive benefit from treatment. These specific findings for AN are consistent with findings for other groups of psychiatric patients suggesting that even with compulsory treatment legally committed patients can derive benefit from treatment and many eventually come to recognize that they did require the involuntary treatment (Kane, Quitkin, Rifkin, Wegner, Rosenberg, & Borenstein, 1983; Kjellin, Andersson, Candefjord, Palmstierna, & Wallsten, 1997).

Impact of anorexia nervosa on others

Experiences of treating anorexia nervosa

The experiences of treating and/or caregiving for patients with anorexia nervosa are among the most challenging of any health problem yet have received relatively little attention. Venables (1930), in a remarkably astute and compassionate early account of the treatment of nine cases of AN, indicated the need for clinicians to exercise patience and emphasized the importance of not losing one's temper when working with such patients. The frustrations and negative reactions evoked by these patients are well known to clinicians (Strober, 2004) and well documented (Morgan, 1977). Dr. Michael Strober, an expert on eating disorders at the UCLA Neuropsychiatric Institute, has written about the particular challenges of managing chronic cases of AN. Strober (2004) notes: "With anorexia nervosa, the challenges are especially daunting because the affliction is maddeningly egosyntonic and neither family nor therapist apprehensions are easily contained" (p. 245).

It is not uncommon for even well-trained, well-meaning clinicians, eager and invested in helping, to experience anxiety when working with dangerously low weight cases and to become frustrated. Such feelings of anxiety and frustration sometimes lead to anger and hostility, especially during moments when the refusal to eat is (mistakenly) simplified to a simple act of rebellion or choice. This is not an unfamiliar occurrence seen even in inpatient services, even in those with experience in treating severe cases of AN. Text Box 3.3 provides some examples of clinical reactions and challenges when working with severe cases of AN.

TEXT BOX 3.3
Examples of common clinical reactions and struggles with hospitalized patients with anorexia nervosa

A typical scenario involves a time-intensive nursing staff intervention to support and encourage a severely underweight patient with AN to eat a small quantity of food following a specified behavioral plan. The psychiatric nurse spends a painstaking hour with the young AN patient encouraging and repeatedly telling her that she is "feeding her brain" and that she will "not get fat from the food." The hour passes, and at least a few bites of food appear to have been tolerated by the patient (even the experienced nurse failed to notice that some of the food was never actually eaten). The nurse attempts to reinforce the patient and encourages her to speak up about her step-by-step progress in a group therapy meeting that is about to begin shortly. A few minutes later, the nurse returns to remind the patient about the group only to discover her exercising frantically in her room after having managed to induce vomiting the moment the nurse had left her. Frustration and anger fill the nurse. During rounds the following morning, another clinician reports on the events of the family therapy meeting and describes the family's hopelessness and resignation over the "loss" of their daughter. The nurse relates to the family's frustrations and reports on the AN patient's behaviors. A debate follows about the specifics of the eating regimen and whether or when to institute more aggressive re-feeding methods.

A second typical scenario involves a frail-looking emaciated young female with AN whose weight has held steady just below 80 pounds. Her behavioral program has been modified over and over again with the view of reinforcing minimal weight gains with additional social privileges and lessened restriction on the inpatient unit. Week after week she fails to gain even the target of 0.5 pounds. She is confronted repeatedly by the clinical staff about her "symptomatic behavior" (i.e., she is asked over and over again about whether she is over-exercising or vomiting or just not really eating the food portions that she seems to eat before leaving the supervised meal table). She responses with much tearfulness (one staff member described her as having "instant crocodile tears") and fierce denial. Increased scrutiny revealed this patient's ability to be constantly in motion without detection (e.g., fidgeting and moving legs under the table or under a blanket to "keep warm"; frenzied brief bouts of exercise in her room when staff were not observing her; sneaking food off her plate into sleeves or pant cuffs). One new staff member, upon discovering her, voiced amazement at the activity level he observed in this person who looked to be near death at other times. Her denial and verbalized puzzlement over not gaining weight or privileges interestingly evoked as much patient criticism (including angry

continues overleaf

TEXT BOX 3.3

continued

outbursts from other patients with eating disorders) as support during the patients' community meetings on the unit. After her eventual discharge after achieving 85 pounds, she shared with a genuinely curious staff some of her various tricks for making or coming close to weight goals on numerous occasions (sticking a couple of batteries in her underwear or taping them to her underarms, not urinating overnight and drinking water before the morning weigh-in).

A third scenario involves an active and heated debate among the staff about whether time is running out before force feeding will be needed to save a male with AN in his early twenties. Several staff members debate the virtues of involuntary feeding for this male patient. One staff member voices his concern about the perceived invasiveness and abusive nature of such interventions. Another staff member recalls a patient asking for such feeding as a way to manage her ambivalence and guilt over her wish to gain weight to live. The unit chief listened quietly as she recalled yesterday's meeting with the patient's mother who tearfully described her images of her son when he was a young and happy boy. The patient's mother was racked by guilt as she described what was best understood as a painful grieving for the loss of her child.

COMMENT

While these are not universal experiences they are also not uncommon examples of some strong clinical challenges and struggles that are well known to clinicians working in inpatient units that provide services to severe cases of AN. It is easy to see from these examples how these frail outwardly passive looking persons can elicit a myriad of potent reactions from clinicians, family members, and even other patients struggling with the same disorder. For a thoughtful discussion of the clinical challenges faced by clinicians who work with severe or chronic forms of AN, the reader is referred to Strober (2004).

Qualitative accounts of carers' experiences

A number of recent qualitative studies of the experience of family members and parents of patients with AN have been recently published (Beale, McMaster, & Hillege, 2005; McMaster, Beale, Hillege, & Nagy, 2004; Treasure, Murphy, Szmukler, Todd, Gavan, & Joyce, 2001). These shed some light on the complex experiences of those who know someone struggling with AN. Such descriptions are also notable in their portrayals of frequent frustrations between families and clinicians. These qualitative analyses of the experiences of caregivers for AN seem to generally convey considerably greater levels of distress than similar qualitative analyses of caregivers for patients with bulimia nervosa (e.g., Perkins, Winn, Murray, Murphy, & Schmidt, 2004; Winn, Perkins, Murray, Murphy, & Schmidt, 2004).

Patients' perspectives

There are many accounts from the patients' perspective of the process of struggling with and in many cases recovering from AN (Weaver, Wuest, & Ciliska, 2005). One such account is told jointly by a mother and daughter about the daughter's AN and recovery (Hughes & Hughes, 2004). There is a large literature of such accounts (e.g., the publisher Gurze Books lists many books describing the lives of children, adolescents, and adults who have had AN. There have also been structured attempts to analyze themes from such literary works written by authors suffering from AN (Stirn, Overbeck, & Pokorny, 2005).

Strober (2004, pp. 245–246) further captured the complexity of treatment for AN when he wrote:

> Even when patient, family, and therapist commit unequivocally to see it through, compassion for the sufferer can quickly reach a limit. As for faith in the therapist's acumen, it too is brittle. It is immaterial to panic-stricken loved ones, or to the well-mannered but quietly seething and mistrustful patient, that from the very beginning the therapist is called on to render decisions of extraordinary delicacy. The slightest misstep, even interventions eminently sensible and vital to the patient's welfare, become flashpoints for angry and entrenched resistance, symptom exacerbation, family antagonism, or abrupt termination of a treatment scarcely begun. When the patient is chronically ill, fear, impotence, and frustration bedevil even the most skilled therapist.

Indeed, this captures the apparent ever-present sense of urgency against a backdrop of the realization that perhaps as many as half of AN patients will have lifelong struggles. In striking contrast is the frequent simplistic view that AN represents little more than an acting-out behavior by an oppositional adolescent girl. Hughes and Hughes (2004), in their poignant description of a daughter's struggles and recovery from AN, documented that when seeking inpatient hospitalization after a series of failed outpatient treatments, a "gatekeeper from the insurance company" refused to approve the hospitalization. Hughes and Hughes (2004) noted that this person "could not understand why we did not just insist that she drink her 'Boost' – a high-calorie liquid supplement" (p. 258).

Experience of family members caring for patients with anorexia nervosa

Until recently, relatively little research has addressed the experience of caregiving by family members to patients with eating disorders. This is surprising since many eating disordered patients are adolescents and still living with their parents. Research on caregiving for a variety of medical and psychiatric problems has generally found that, despite some positive aspects, caregivers frequently experience high levels of stress and burden and can benefit from support (Szmukler, Wykes, & Parkman, 1998). The little research conducted to date with caregivers of AN has revealed the very significant burden and stress associated with helping family members with this specific problem.

In a preliminary study, Santonastaso, Saccon, and Favaro (1997) assessed 40 relatives of 24 patients with eating disorders. The relatives of patients with AN reported significantly higher subjective burden of caregiving than did the relatives of patients with BN. This study also found that the relatives of AN patients reported greater psychiatric symptoms and seemed to be overinvolved compared to the relatives of BN patients.

More recently, Janet Treasure and her colleagues (2001), in a study conducted in the United Kingdom, compared 71 relatives who provided care to patients with AN to 68 relatives who provided care to persons with psychotic illnesses. For the AN caregivers, 60% were parents, 12% were siblings, 16% were spouses, and the remaining 12% did not specify the relationship. Although the AN patients were younger than the psychotic patients, the duration of the illnesses was similar, which allowed for a reasonable comparison of the caregiving experience. Overall, the caregivers of the AN patients reported significantly more overall difficulties with caring for the patients than did the caregivers of patients with psychotic illnesses. Inspection of the specific areas of difficulties voiced by the caregivers of the AN and psychotic patients did not reveal significant differences although there were consistent trends for greater concerns being voiced by the AN caregivers for difficult behaviors and negative symptoms, stigma, effects on the family, dependency and loss issues, and problems with clinical services. The caregivers of AN patients reported significantly higher general psychological distress as a result than did the caregivers of patients with psychotic illnesses. Analyses revealed that specific concerns about the AN patients' "difficult behaviors," "negative symptoms," "loss," and problems with clinical services were related to the heightened distress.

Summary

Anorexia nervosa is characterized by the refusal to maintain a minimal body weight, extreme food restriction and weight control behaviors, and an intense fear of fat or weight gain despite a seriously underweight condition. AN is frequently not viewed as a problem by those afflicted with it who view their ability to severely restrict eating and control weight as highly desirable. Patients with AN are frequently obsessional and perfectionistic, a combination that along with a typically remarkable degree of denial about their problem results in a truly challenging problem for clinicians and caregivers. AN is associated with high rates of medical problems and still has one of the highest death rates of any psychiatric problem. The perplexing nature of AN has been a challenge to clinical researchers and limited progress has been achieved either in understanding or treating AN. AN remains a frequently chronic and debilitating disorder with most studies finding that 50% of patients do not recover even after long periods of time and numerous treatments.

Understanding, assessing, and treating bulimia nervosa 4

Introduction

Bulimia nervosa (BN) has been the focus of aggressive research efforts since Russell's (1979) paper describing bulimia nervosa. The striking convergence of several descriptive accounts of bulimia nervosa that soon followed from several countries stimulated research on this problem (Abraham & Beumont, 1982; Fairburn & Cooper, 1982; Pyle et al., 1981). In the two decades that followed, considerable progress has been achieved. As noted in chapter 2, there remains uncertainty about the exact nature of the distribution of BN and very little is known about its etiology or development. Thus, additional research is necessary to inform how to proceed with prevention or early intervention programs. In contrast, progress has been made in understanding factors that serve to maintain the disorder. This, in turn, has resulted in considerable progress in establishing the utility of certain treatments. Text Box 4.1 gives some clinical examples of bulimia nervosa. The chapter then continues with an overview of the major assessment issues relevant to BN followed by a summary of the major research findings about treatments.

Assessment of bulimia nervosa

The assessment of BN is complicated by a number of factors. First, many persons with BN are tremendously embarrassed and ashamed about their problem and are frequently unwilling to reveal it. The secrecy frequently goes beyond just shame. For instance, in many instances when friends, family, or even health care providers inquire about these problems, persons with BN will deny the problem. This denial is very different from the denial characteristic of many persons with anorexia nervosa (AN). In AN, the denial of the

TEXT BOX 4.1

Clinical examples of bulimia nervosa

J.S. is a 19-year-old single white female. She had always been average weight but tended to feel slightly overweight. During her freshman year in college she gained 25 pounds. When she returned home for the summer, she felt a bit uncomfortable wearing light clothes. Within a week's time she either perceived or was the recipient of several unkind teasing comments from several peers and an unsupportive comment from her mother. She decided to diet and began to decrease her eating and began to exercise. She returned to college ten pounds lighter and continued to diet reasonably. Several of her peers living in her dorm suite had also begun to diet during the summer and they all began to share their experiences and to try to support each other.

The hectic schedule and high stress were making it difficult for J.S. to stick to her plan. She found herself overeating frequently and trying to "make up for the calories" by skipping meals, particularly during the morning and afternoon. She soon found herself gaining a little bit of weight while a few of her friends were losing weight. She resolved to try harder and set up a stricter diet plan. One Friday, after a very tough and upsetting day, she suddenly found herself eating everything she could get her hands on. She ate uncontrollably until she ran out of food and found herself physically distressed. This pattern repeated itself for about a month at which time she learned that one of her peers had also been binge eating but she had learned to self-induce vomiting after eating. It took J.S. several attempts, but she was soon able to self-induce vomiting after binge eating. This pattern escalated and by the time J.S. went home for summer vacation, she was binge eating and vomiting several times per week. These episodes of loss of control alternated with other periods during which she strictly controlled her eating.

T.M. was another one of the girls in this dorm. She was a student-athlete and competed on the track team doing cross-country. She had always been an athlete and thin. As a girl she was a dancer but she took up running when she felt unable to compete with her peers who were dancers but were naturally even thinner than she was (she was quite lean). She soon became very engrossed in her running. She delighted in the long periods of solitude and in the sense of accomplishment and control she experienced by tightly controlling her weight while successfully competing. She started off thinner than the other girls in the dorm and typically ate far less than them. During a stressful second semester, she experienced several situations in which she allowed herself to overeat and even engaged in what seemed to be group binge eating sessions. She experienced powerful mixed feelings about this and it went on for about two to three months. During this time, she intensified her running as a means to compensate for the overeating. During her running, she resolved to "take back control" of her eating. For the next two months she severely cut her food intake while increasing her running. She essentially ate minimal protein (white tuna fish) and vegetables and little else. Initially she received praise from others, who did not understand the extent or severity of her situation. This soon turned to concern by others, but she simply denied it. She went home for the summer at a weight of 90 pounds. She did not return to college the following year.

COMMENTS

These examples reflect clinical presentations commonly seen in patients with BN. Although they reflect different genders, age periods, methods of extreme weight control, and courses of illness, they are readily understood with a general cognitive behavioral model of maintenance.

continues

Sociocultural pressures to achieve a particular weight goal or shape impact on certain susceptible individuals. The exact nature of this vulnerability is uncertain, but likely reflects multiple factors, including genetic and familial predispositions, psychological factors including poor self-esteem, difficulties with emotional distress or regulation, and certain cognitive styles such as perfectionistic tendencies. Dieting to control weight begins but is insufficiently successful and this leads to more extreme dietary restriction (such as skipping meals) and this physiological and psychological deprivation sets the stage for binge eating. Binge eating fuels concerns regarding weight and shape and leads to even stricter attempts to restrict eating, which in turn inevitably triggers binge eating.

Some individuals learn of extreme weight control practices and begin to use them to cope with the distress of the binge eating. Most commonly, patients with BN self-induce vomiting, although other methods such as laxative abuse, and misuse of diet pill and diuretics are used. Extreme exercise is used by some patients either in combination with purging or as a primary method to purge.

The first case (J.S.) represents a prototypic example of bulimia nervosa. In contrast, the second case provided above (T.M.) represents a female with a likely history of anorexia nervosa who years later briefly developed bulimic symptoms before succumbing to a clear episode of anorexia nervosa.

problem reflects the nature of the disorder (for example, the low weight or restricted eating are viewed by the patient as achievements, not problems). In BN, the person is distressed by the symptoms and greatly concerned by the behaviors. However, they are ambivalent about disclosing the problem or pursuing treatment. This is because the overvalued ideas regarding weight and shape result in the continued goal of becoming a better dieter. Until the individual with BN achieves the elusive goal of "optimal dietary control" they have the belief that the purging behaviors are at least effective for controlling their weight.

Second, many persons with BN are approximately of average weight and are able to hide their eating disorder. There are very few observable physical signs, most persons with BN will have normal laboratory tests (Greenfeld, Mickley, Quinlan, & Roloff, 1995), and while they are still young they frequently do not manifest physical signs and symptoms until the disorder worsens. This is unfortunate because BN is associated with considerable medical problems (described later).

Third, persons with BN frequently have problems with social relatedness and interpersonal relations (Herzog, Keller, Lavori, & Ott, 1988; Johnson & Connors, 1987). These interpersonal deficits interfere with their ability to obtain and make use of social support or help from others. These social deficits combine with their intense preoccupation with physical appearance to make the individual exquisitely sensitive to how others might perceive them. Persons with BN often have high levels of public self-consciousness and social anxiety and strive very hard to come across as healthy as possible (Striegel-Moore, Silberstein, & Rodin, 1993). They try to appear as competent as possible and behave in accordance with how they believe others want them to. Thus, many persons with BN will appear outwardly competent and successful and will work hard to hide their perceived faults and problems, including the BN, from others.

Assessment measures

The same structured interviews described in chapter 3 are also relevant for BN. The EDE interview (Fairburn & Cooper, 1993) is widely used in studies with BN and regarded by some as the best method for characterizing the features of eating disorders. As noted earlier, self-report inventories offer easier and less costly means of obtaining important information and offer a good solution when expert interviewers are not available or when screening (rather than diagnosis) is the goal. The reader is referred to Grilo (2005) for a detailed discussion of these issues and detailed discussion of different methods. In terms of self-report instruments, the EDE-Q has received good support for use with BN patients (Black & Wilson, 1996; Carter, Aime, & Mills, 2001; Mond, Hay, Rodgers, Owen, & Beumont, 2004; Sysko, Walsh, & Fairburn, 2005). The study by Sysko and colleagues (2005) specifically demonstrated the utility of the EDE-Q for assessing change and outcome in patients with BN; the EDE-Q and EDE interview yielded comparable findings in patterns of changes in bulimic symptomatology. In general, such studies suggest that self-report methods may be somewhat more useful in patients with BN than AN and for assessing certain behavioral features such as purging.

Medical assessment and co-morbidities

Although less dangerous than anorexia nervosa, medical complications are not uncommon in BN (APA, 2000b; Pomeroy & Mitchell, 1996). The medical complications can occur due to the extreme dieting, binge eating, and purging behaviors. In general, a combination of lower weight and higher purging is associated with greater

TABLE 4.1

Common physical and medical issues associated with bulimia nervosa

Renal and electrolyte problems
- Electrolyte abnormalities and disrupted fluid homeostasis are common in purging bulimics and in underweight severely restricting patients. Most common serious electrolyte abnormality is hypokalemia (potassium loss).
- Hypovolemic state can occur in those who purge frequently.

Cardiovascular system
- Abnormalities most common in patients with electrolyte abnormalities. In such cases, serious cardiac arrhythmias and conduction deficits can occur and require immediate attention.
- High concern among (rare) ipecac abusers.
- Hypotension common due to dehydration from purging.

Gastrointestinal system
- Every portion of gastrointestinal (GI) tract can be influenced.
- Salivary glands are often enlarged (note: this is important and one of the few helpful physical signs to signal possible BN).
- Esophageal problems (gastritis, esophagitis, bleeding, gastric tears).
- Loss of normal peristaltic function (frequent complaints of GI cramps and intermixed diarrhea and constipation) common in laxative abusers.

Endocrine system
- Endocrine abnormalities seen in anorexia nervosa are less common or severe in BN.

Dental system
- Dental damage is a major common problem in BN. Dental decay or erosion is common among BN patients who regularly induce vomiting.

Dermatological system
- Calluses, abrasions, or bruises on the hands or thumbs (Russell's sign) signal recurrent self-induced vomiting.

Reproductive system
- Increased rates of miscarriage and obstetrical problems exist in BN.
- Babies frequently have low weight.

medical risk. Table 4.1 summarizes the major body systems that are influenced by BN and the most common medical concerns with these patients.

A comprehensive listing of laboratory tests that can be used to assess common physical complications of bulimia nervosa across the most vulnerable organ systems can be found in the *Revised Practice Guidelines for the Treatment of Patients With Eating Disorders* published by the American Psychiatric Association (2000b).

Psychological assessment

As noted previously in chapter 2 for anorexia nervosa, it is important to assess the other major psychiatric or psychological problems that may be present in persons with BN. Indeed, BN is associated with high rates of other psychiatric problems and psychological distress. The exact nature and significance of co-occurring psychiatric problems remains uncertain. For example, different problems may co-occur ("co-morbidity") for a variety of reasons. These may include various shared underlying causes, a third factor causes the two problems, one problem causes the other problem, or simply that two unrelated problems can occur in a person over time. A general finding is that community samples of persons with BN have fewer co-occurring problems than outpatient samples which in turn have fewer associated problems than inpatient groups. Thus, higher rates of co-occurring problems may reflect greater severity in the eating disorder or greater psychiatric difficulties in general. Elevated rates of associated problems may also reflect various sampling confounds and biases characteristic of treatment-seeking patients that make interpretation of these findings difficult (Fairburn et al., 1996). Although the exact meaning of co-occurring psychiatric problems for understanding the underlying nature of BN is uncertain, it is important to determine the presence of other problems. This is essential for good clinical management and for prioritizing treatments.

Certain psychiatric problems are particularly common in patients with BN, most notably depression, anxiety, and substance abuse (Grilo et al., 1995a, 1995b; Grilo et al., 1996; Schwalberg, Barlow, Alger, & Howard, 1992), and certain forms of personality disorders (Grilo et al., 2003b). Many studies with clinical samples report that as many as 80% of BN patients have at least one additional psychiatric disorder over their lifetime (Fichter & Quadflieg, 1997). The most commonly associated problem are the mood disorders, with most studies reporting roughly 50% lifetime rate of major depressive disorder in patients with BN. Across studies that have used well-established assessment instruments, rates of major depressive disorder are generally between 30% in community samples and 65% in inpatient samples. Anxiety disorders are also common but rates range markedly (10% to 65%) across studies (Herzog et al., 1992), with social phobia and obsessive-compulsive disorder the most commonly seen forms of anxiety disorders in BN (Brewerton, Lydiard, Herzog, Brotman, O'Neil, & Ballenger, 1995a; Von Ranson, Kaye, Weltzin, Rao,

& Matsunaga, 1999). Studies generally report that roughly one-fourth of patients with BN have substance use disorders (Bulik et al., 1994). BN patients with co-occurring substance abuse are most likely to have borderline personality disorder and heightened levels of impulsivity (Grilo et al., 1995a) and engage in various self-destructive and injurious behaviors (Bulik et al., 1994). Research has found considerable variability in the temporal sequence of when BN patients develop these other psychiatric problems. Research has found that the onset of co-occurring problems sometimes occurs before, sometimes concurrent with, and sometimes after BN develops. More specifically, findings suggest anxiety disorders more frequently precede BN and substance use disorders more frequently follow BN (Braun et al., 1994).

Overview of treatments for bulimia nervosa

In contrast to the limited research on the treatment of anorexia nervosa, the past 20 years have witnessed the rapid development of pharmacological and psychological treatments for BN. Over 60 randomized controlled trials with BN have been performed. This research has found considerable differences in the effectiveness of specific treatments allowing for clear conclusions and treatment guidelines to be suggested. Unlike the case for AN, the prognosis for patients with BN who receive the best available treatments is good. Roughly 50% of patients with BN who receive manual-based cognitive behavioral therapy (CBT; a specific structured form of psychotherapy) achieve either near or full recovery that appears to be well-maintained over time. A brief overview of what is known about the treatment of BN follows. This discussion will selectively address the major research findings since there is a fair amount of expert consensus.

Pharmacotherapy

The vast majority of pharmacotherapy studies for BN have tested antidepressant medications. This approach was initially stimulated by clinical observations that many patients with BN had histories of depression and the view that this eating disorder might represent a variant of depression (Hudson, Pope, Jonas, & Yurgelun-Todd, 1983). Subsequent research has not supported the view that BN is a form of depression. Interestingly, although antidepressants produce improvements in some patients with BN, positive response is not predicted by the presence of history of depression. A few studies have tested other classes of medications without notable success.

Antidepressant medication is frequently reported to be statistically superior to placebo conditions in controlled trials (e.g., fluoxetine; FBNCSG, 1992; Goldstein, Wilson, Thompson, Potvin, & Rampey, 1995). Meta-analyses, however, conclude that there is limited evidence suggesting a clinically significant difference between pharmacotherapy and placebo with antidepressants being superior (Bacaltchuk & Hay, 2003; NICE, 2004).

The recent Cochrane Collaborative meta-analysis of randomized controlled studies of antidepressants for BN (Bacaltchuk & Hay, 2003) considered ten studies that met certain quality requirements. Overall, across these ten studies, remission (defined as one week without binge eating or purging) was observed in 19% of patients receiving antidepressant medication versus 8% of patients receiving placebo. While many of those individual studies reported statistically significant advantage for the medication over placebo, the meta-analysis by Bacaltchuk and Hay (2003) reveals an effect size suggesting the effects are modest from a clinical perspective. These findings are summarized in Figure 4.1. The relative risk ratio of 0.88 suggests that medication reduced the risk of not remitting by 12%. A separate carefully conducted meta-analysis performed by NICE (2004) which included only six studies based on their quality requirements, resulted in essentially the same findings (relative risk ratio of 0.88) and conclusions.

There are two concerns about pharmacotherapy that must also be considered although they are frequently overlooked. First, most pharmacotherapy research on BN has been of relatively short duration and often follow-up data has not been obtained. Thus, little is known about how long to treat patients with medication or how durable the effects of medication are if discontinued. The few available data suggest that relapse in BN is frequent after patients discontinue medications (Agras, 1997; Walsh, Hadigan, Devlin, Gladis, & Roose, 1991). Second, although pharmacotherapy reduces binge eating, it does not seem to decrease the extreme dietary restriction characteristic of BN (Craighead & Agras, 1991). Thus, a core behavioral symptom of BN is not alleviated and, in fact, may be strengthened (i.e., helping the BN to become a "stronger dieter") by these

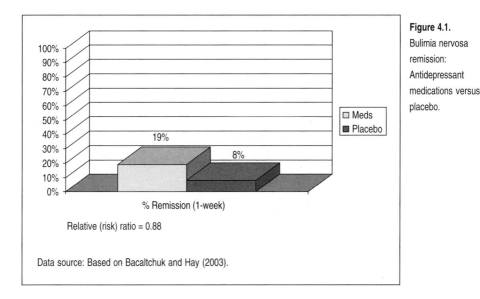

Figure 4.1.
Bulimia nervosa remission: Antidepressant medications versus placebo.

medications. This may contribute to the short-term decrease in binge eating observed. However, the heightened unhealthy dietary restraint will eventually fail and lead to repeated binge eating.

Cognitive behavioral therapy (CBT) and psychological approaches for BN

CBT versus controls

Qualitative reviews (Wilson, 2005), quantitative analyses (Hay et al., 2004; Whittal, Agras, & Gould, 1999), and expert consensus (Grilo, Devlin, Cachelin, & Yanovski, 1997; Fairburn & Harrison, 2003; Wilson & Shafran, 2005) conclude that CBT is the treatment of choice for bulimia nervosa. The recent Cochrane Collaborative meta-analysis of randomized controlled studies of CBT versus wait-list or control conditions for BN (Hay et al., 2004) considered eight studies that met certain quality requirements. Overall, across these studies, remission (defined as four weeks without binge eating or purging) was observed in 40% of patients receiving CBT versus 5% in patients in control conditions. These findings are summarized in Figure 4.2. These findings suggest that robust and clinically-meaningful improvements are produced by CBT.

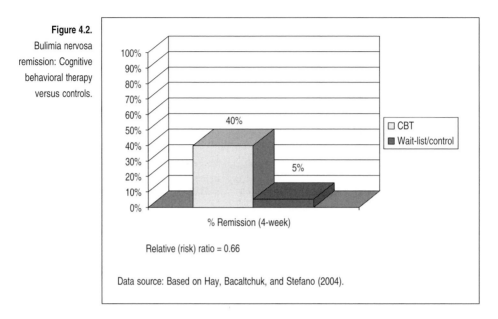

Relative (risk) ratio = 0.66

Data source: Based on Hay, Bacaltchuk, and Stefano (2004).

In contrast to pharmacotherapy treatments, CBT for BN typically reduces the excessive dietary restriction seen in these patients. Thus, the desired reductions in binge eating and purging are achieved in conjunction with normalized and healthier eating patterns. Wilson, Fairburn, Agras, Walsh, & Kraemer (2002) demonstrated that these reductions in dietary restriction played an important role in decreasing binge eating.

CBT versus alternative psychotherapies

CBT has been generally found to be significantly superior to several other psychological treatments in diverse controlled treatment studies. CBT was superior to non-directive group psychotherapy (Kirkley, Schneider, Agras, & Bachman, 1985), supportive-expressive therapy (Garner, Rockert, Davis, Garner, Olmsted, & Eagle, 1993; Walsh et al., 1997), behavior therapy (Fairburn et al., 1991, 1993a, 1993b), and interpersonal psychotherapy (Agras et al., 2000).

Figure 4.3 summarizes the treatment outcomes from a controlled trial performed at Oxford University comparing three different psychological treatments for BN. Fairburn and colleagues randomly assigned 75 consecutive BN patients to one of three treatments: behavioral therapy (BT), cognitive behavioral therapy (CBT), or interpersonal psychotherapy (IPT). The treatments were provided in 19

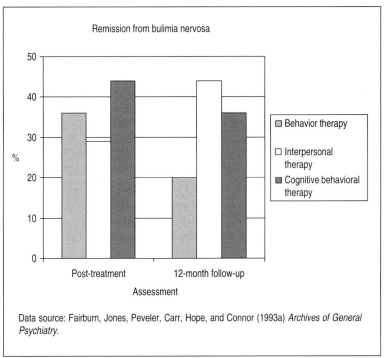

Figure 4.3.

Three psychotherapies for bulimia nervosa.

Remission from bulimia nervosa

50

40

%

30

20

10

0

Post-treatment   12-month follow-up

Assessment

☐ Behavior therapy

☐ Interpersonal therapy

■ Cognitive behavioral therapy

Data source: Fairburn, Jones, Peveler, Carr, Hope, and Connor (1993a) *Archives of General Psychiatry.*

individual sessions over 18 weeks. Figure 4.3 shows the outcomes at the end of treatment (Fairburn et al., 1991) and at a follow-up conducted 12 months later (Fairburn et al., 1993a). All three treatments resulted in significant and comparable improvements in binge eating and purging by the end of treatment (left side of Figure 4.3). CBT resulted in greater improvements in the overvalued ideas regarding shape and weight than both the BT and IPT. At 12-month follow-up, however, there were striking differences between the treatments (right side of Figure 4.3). Whereas BT was associated with a return of problems, patients in the CBT and IPT treatments achieved significant and comparable levels of lasting clinical improvements.

The study by Fairburn and colleagues (1993a) was especially noteworthy in finding an alternative therapy (IPT) to CBT that achieved comparable and lasting improvements. This is interesting because it raised the possibility that BN could be treated successfully without direct focus on eating habits or cognitions about shape and weight. Interpersonal psychotherapy is a focal therapy that addresses interpersonal deficits. See Table 4.2 for a comparison of CBT and IPT for BN (and more generally for binge eating disorder, which will be

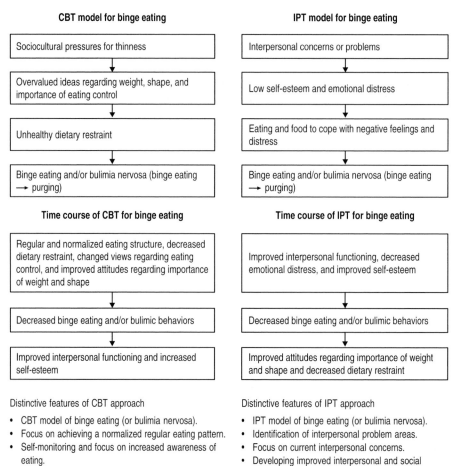

TABLE 4.2

Comparison of cognitive behavioral therapy (CBT) and interpersonal psychotherapy (IPT) for binge eating problems (bulimia nervosa and binge eating disorder)

CBT model for binge eating

Sociocultural pressures for thinness

↓

Overvalued ideas regarding weight, shape, and importance of eating control

↓

Unhealthy dietary restraint

↓

Binge eating and/or bulimia nervosa (binge eating ⟶ purging)

IPT model for binge eating

Interpersonal concerns or problems

↓

Low self-esteem and emotional distress

↓

Eating and food to cope with negative feelings and distress

↓

Binge eating and/or bulimia nervosa (binge eating ⟶ purging)

Time course of CBT for binge eating

Regular and normalized eating structure, decreased dietary restraint, changed views regarding eating control, and improved attitudes regarding importance of weight and shape

↓

Decreased binge eating and/or bulimic behaviors

↓

Improved interpersonal functioning and increased self-esteem

Time course of IPT for binge eating

Improved interpersonal functioning, decreased emotional distress, and improved self-esteem

↓

Decreased binge eating and/or bulimic behaviors

↓

Improved attitudes regarding importance of weight and shape and decreased dietary restraint

Distinctive features of CBT approach

- CBT model of binge eating (or bulimia nervosa).
- Focus on achieving a normalized regular eating pattern.
- Self-monitoring and focus on increased awareness of eating.
- Identifying and modifying distorted attitudes regarding weight/shape.
- Coping skills for triggers of binge eating (and bulimic behaviors).
- Relapse prevention (how to deal with setbacks).

Distinctive features of IPT approach

- IPT model of binge eating (or bulimia nervosa).
- Identification of interpersonal problem areas.
- Focus on current interpersonal concerns.
- Developing improved interpersonal and social skills.
- Tolerance and exploration of emotions.
- Termination of treatment as example of separation or loss.

This summary comparing CBT versus IPT is based on detailed descriptions of CBT (Fairburn et al., 1993b; Wilson, Fairburn, & Agras, 1997) and IPT (Fairburn, 1997; Wilfley, MacKenzie, Welch, Ayes, & Weissman, 2000) for both binge eating and bulimia nervosa. This summary is adapted from a detailed comparison of CBT and IPT (Wilfley, Grilo, & Rodin, 1997). The interested reader is referred to Wilfley and colleagues (1997) for a detailed description of the assessment and intervention stages and procedures for both of these treatments.

discussed in chapter 5). The interested reader is referred to a detailed description of the conceptual model of IPT for BN (Fairburn, 1997) and to the therapy manual provided by Wilfley et al. (1997) and Wilfley, MacKenzie, Welch, Ayes, and Weissman (2000).

More recently, a larger multi-site study found that CBT was significantly superior to IPT for the treatment of BN and achieved its effects more rapidly (Agras et al., 2000a). Agras and colleagues (2000a) reported that CBT resulted in a significantly higher "recovery" rate (no binge eating or purging for a month) than IPT at the end of treatment (29% versus 6%). Interestingly, at 12-month follow-up, the reported recovery rates for CBT and IPT no longer differed significantly. The authors concluded that collectively these findings (notably the faster improvement by CBT) suggest that CBT be considered the treatment of choice for BN.

Psychological and/or pharmacological treatments

Controlled studies that have included direct comparisons of CBT and pharmacotherapy have consistently found that CBT alone is superior to medication alone (Goldbloom et al., 1997; Leitenberg, Rosen, Wolf, Vara, Detzer, & Srebnik, 1994; Mitchell, Pyle, Eckert, Hatsukami, Pomeroy, & Zimmerman, 1990; Walsh et al., 1997). A combination of antidepressant treatment and CBT is superior to antidepressant treatment alone (Agras et al., 1992; Goldbloom et al., 1997; Leitenberg et al., 1994; Mitchell et al., 1990; Walsh et al., 1997) but is generally comparable to CBT alone (Agras et al., 1992; Fichter, Leibl, Rief, Brunner, Schmidt-Auberger, & Engel, 1991; Goldbloom et al., 1997). Two studies, though, reported a slight advantage for the combination for some symptoms (Mitchell et al., 1990; Walsh et al., 1997).

Self-help forms of cognitive behavioral therapy

Many compelling reasons exist for developing and testing self-help programs for eating disorders for use by persons who are interested or motivated to change. First, although certain forms of treatment such as CBT appear to be effective when delivered by specialized clinicians, there are many places that lack therapists with training in these specific methods. Even when there is adequate availability of clinical services, there exist barriers to treatment. Persons with bulimia nervosa – in spite of its seriousness – seek treatment less frequently than individuals with other psychiatric disorders (Whitaker et al., 1990). The majority of persons with BN do not seek treatment for a variety of reasons. One reason might be ambivalence towards altering their behavior. Other reasons may range from practical (lack of insurance or financial resources to pay for treatment) to strong feelings of embarrassment and shame about these problems that serve to keep them private and secretive. Self-help programs, if effective, could potentially represent a valuable resource in these types of situations.

Grilo (2000), in a review of adaptations of CBT for guided self-help (CBTgsh) and pure self-help (CBTsh) methods of administration, noted that a number of studies conducted in the US and Europe found that some of these treatments were significantly superior to control conditions for BN (e.g., Cooper, Coker, & Fleming, 1996; Mitchell et al., 2001; Thiels, Schmidt, Treasure, Garthe, & Troop, 1998; Treasure, Schmidt, Troop, Tiller, Todd, & Turnbull, 1996). Collectively, these controlled studies found both short-term and longer term efficacy (i.e., good maintenance at follow-up evaluations after treatment discontinuation). The efficacy of such self-help adaptations of CBT for BN have received additional support in subsequent controlled trials (Carter, Olmstead, Kaplan, McCabe, Mills, & Aime, 2003; Mitchell et al., 2001; Palmer, Birchall, McGrain, & Sullivan, 2002).

Although these CBT adaptations have the obvious potential for wider dissemination, further investigation is necessary as research to date has resulted in mixed findings. A recent randomized controlled study in England for BN (Durand & King, 2003) found that CBTgsh administered in general practice and CBT administered in a specialist eating disorder clinic both produced substantial improvements that did not differ significantly by condition. Bailer and colleagues (2004) found that CBTgsh and group CBT resulted in comparable and significant improvements that were reasonably well sustained at one-year follow-up. These positive outcomes were achieved by relatively inexperienced psychiatric residents. In sharp contrast, in a study performed in a primary care setting, Walsh, Fairburn, Mickley, Sysko, and Parides (2004) reported that CBTgsh given by nurses had a very high dropout rate and resulted in very little clinical improvement. In this specific primary care setting, pharmacotherapy with fluoxetine was associated with better retention and greater clinical improvement than the CBTgsh (Walsh et al., 2004).

The findings by Walsh et al. (2004) for BN patients in primary care are in sharp contrast to those reported by Mitchell and colleagues (2001) using the same exact study design in a specialized eating disorder clinic. Mitchell et al. (2001) reported substantially higher treatment completion rates and better clinical outcomes for both CBTsh and for fluoxetine in the specialized centers than reported by Walsh et al. (2004) for the primary care settings. In the Mitchell et al. (2001) study, both CBTsh and fluoxetine were found to be effective and the two treatments had a significant additive effect. Continued research is needed to determine how best to disseminate these treatments.

What is cognitive behavioral therapy (CBT)?

Given the consistent and robust support for CBT as the treatment of choice for BN (NICE, 2004), a description follows. CBT for BN is based on a clear cognitive model of the maintenance of this eating disorder. This cognitive model views the core psychopathology of BN as the overevaluation of shape and weight. As detailed in chapter 2, these overvalued and dysfunctional concerns drive the extreme dieting and weight loss behaviors. Importantly, the overvalued ideas are reinforced by the behaviors each time they occur. This results in a vicious self-maintaining cycle. Restrictive dieting behaviors (unhealthy "dietary restraint") make individuals vulnerable to binge eating (experience loss of control during overeating). The binge eating, in turn, produces intense physical discomfort or emotional distress and fear of weight gain. The feelings of discomfort and distress, in combination with heightened concerns about shape and weight prompt the purging (self-induced vomiting) or other extreme forms of weight control behaviors (laxative abuse, taking diuretics, abusing diet pills, extreme exercise). After the purging, the individual with BN "recommits" to restrictive dieting, and the cycle repeats.

CBT for BN is a manual-based therapy that systematically addresses each of the components of the BN cycle. CBT is a directive, active, problem-oriented collaborative approach focused on the "here and now." In general, the CBT is provided in 16 to 20 sessions over a four-month period. A detailed manual of the most studied and best established CBT for BN is available (Fairburn et al., 1993b). In addition, the reader is referred to the descriptions by Wilson and colleagues (1997) and by Wilfley et al. (1997) for elaborations of some of the CBT procedures. The description by Wilfley et al. (1997) includes a discussion of broader application of the CBT to binge eating problems (such as BED; see chapter 5) and includes a detailed discussion of the rationale and modification for group therapy methods. This CBT has been most widely studied in individual formats but has also received considerable support in group therapy formats (see Wilfley et al., 1997 for rationale and modifications).

CBT for BN (Fairburn et al., 1993b; Wilson et al., 1997) has three basic stages. The first stage of treatment includes describing and explaining the cognitive behavioral model and demonstrating how it applies to the individual's circumstances. This is followed by a discussion of the structure, goals, interventions, and expected outcomes of the treatment. Information and education is provided about dieting, binge eating, purging and other extreme weight control methods, and their impact on health. This serves to normalize many patients' concerns while correcting many incorrect notions about eating and weight. A critical element of CBT is the introduction of self-monitoring techniques. Self-monitoring refers to detailed record keeping of important behaviors and problems that occur throughout the week (in between the therapy sessions). In this case, self-monitoring involves the recording of all eating behaviors (meals, snacks, binge eating) and associated factors (time of day, setting, hunger, all the food eaten, and any important associated factors such as emotions, triggers, and so forth. Self-monitoring is viewed as the hallmark of CBT and is essential for success. Text Box 4.2 describes self-monitoring and Text Box 4.3 provides an example of self-monitoring.

Behaviorally, the first stage, in addition to the self-monitoring, introduces graded techniques that focus on helping the person to establish normalized regular eating patterns. Most frequently, the patient is encouraged to work towards a structure of three healthy meals and two or three snacks per day. This is critical to break the pattern of restrictive dieting and meal skipping in order to eliminate the episodic binge eating. During this stage, coping methods are also taught to deal with emotional distress and to overcome urges to purge.

The second stage of treatment consists of maintaining the normalized and regular eating patterns and ongoing self-monitoring procedures but becomes increasingly cognitively oriented. Developing alternative coping skills for the triggers of the maladaptive eating patterns and for negative affective states continues to be a focus.

TEXT BOX 4.2
Self-monitoring

Self-monitoring refers to detailed record keeping of important behaviors and problems. Self-monitoring is viewed as the hallmark of CBT and is essential for success. In the case of BN, patients are asked to record all eating behaviors on self-monitoring forms, such as the one shown in Text Box 4.3. Although these forms can vary somewhat, it is important that the patient write down everything they eat along with additional details including: the time of the day; the setting or location; whether it was a meal, snack, or binge eating episode; associated activities, thoughts, feelings, or possible triggers; and whether purging occurred, and if so by what means.

The critical importance of self-monitoring for success is emphasized to patients. This includes a thorough explanation of why self-monitoring is important and how it will be used by *both* the therapist and the patient. The self-monitoring provides a detailed and organized assessment of the eating patterns for the time period between session. Quick inspection provides rich information about the eating patterns. For example, did the patient make any progress towards achieving a regular pattern of eating meals and snacks (rather than strict dieting and skipping meals)? How many binge eating episodes and purging behaviors occurred? If binge eating occurred, was there any patterning (e.g., they happened late in the evening when alone and hungry after not eating all day) or triggers (e.g., emotionally upsetting situations; loneliness)?

Self-monitoring is also a powerful tool for increasing the patient's self-awareness of the binge eating and all of the associated factors. Patients are strongly encouraged to do the record keeping as close to or as soon as possible after the eating occurs, rather than waiting until the end of the day (or the day before the therapy session). This is essential for providing the therapist with accurate and specific information rather than impressionistic and global information that has been clouded by the passage of time. Equally importantly, by learning to do the record keeping as close as possible to the eating, patients begin to increase their self-awareness of both the eating behaviors and possible triggers for the loss of control. Although this is initially uncomfortable and embarrassing for some patients, with support and encouragement, the self-monitoring increases self-awareness, which in turn soon becomes a means to feeling greater control. Invariably, this leads to an important shift in which the patient can see the chain of events unfold rather than just experience the binge–purge behaviors seemingly as a blur happening to them.

Cognitive restructuring is introduced and becomes the major focus of therapy. This portion of treatment pays careful attention to identifying and challenging the maladaptive cognitions and the over-evaluation of shape and weight. Text Box 4.4 provides a detailed description of cognitive restructuring along with a clinical example.

The third stage focuses on the consolidation of progress and on successful maintenance of change post-treatment. "Relapse prevention" techniques are taught. Patients are taught how to identify high-risk situations, perform appropriate coping, and how to manage lapses or return of symptoms or setbacks. The third stage takes a forward-looking stance and includes the focus of continued normalization of eating over time.

TEXT BOX 4.3
Daily self-monitoring and food record

Name: _____   Date: _____

Time of day (Time eating began and ended)	Type and quantity of food (provide as much detail as possible)	M = Meal S = Snack B = Binge	Setting (location, activity and others present)	Purging (how? how many times?)	Thoughts/feelings comments	Pre-meal hunger 0 = no hunger 10 = starving
8:30 a.m.	Apple	Meal	Room		I have to eat something ... this won't be too bad	6
9:00 p.m.					My housemates asked me to go with them to Frank's ... the local pizza shop to hang out. I really wanted to go but I was afraid to go because I'd end up eating pizza and drinking beer. I couldn't do that ... I couldn't handle their comments about how I'm so good ... or worse, if I ended up eating, how I'm so lucky to be able to eat and not be fat.	10
10:00 p.m.	Chicken Caesar wrap and two orders of French fries (pre-pared foods counter)	Binge	Went to the local store and came back to the house		I was so lonely and getting more and more sad and angry.	
	2 large packages of cookies					
	Half pint chocolate ice cream					
	Half of a muffin (left over)				Disgusted and grossed out.	
	Piece of bread			Vomit 2 times	I hate myself. I have to stop doing this	

COMMENTS

This is a sample of a completed self-monitoring record from a 24-year-old single woman sharing a house with several peers who are also attending professional schools at a nearby university. This self-monitoring record covers just one day and was from the third week of treatment. During this particular week, she had three days during which she reported having had a total of four episodes of binge eating and having self-induced vomiting six times. By the third week, she had made substantial progress in several areas.

First, in the important domain of self-monitoring, after first struggling quite a bit with record keeping, she quickly became very good at keeping detailed records. Initially, she skipped record keeping on some days and had great trouble and discomfort with trying to identify and articulate her thoughts and feelings that preceded and followed her binge eating and purging behaviors. She responded well to the support and encouragement given about both the difficulty and the importance of the record keeping. She also found the review and summary of the records by the therapist to be enlightening and helpful. She was also beginning to appreciate the intended benefits of increased awareness. She found herself more frequently self-aware and observant of her ongoing eating and, importantly, her temptations to skip meals. Inspection of the food record above by the therapist revealed something that she was increasingly cognizant of. On this day, she severely restricted her eating the entire day and this set the stage for the binge eating. The dietary restriction made her physiologically deprived and vulnerable to overeating. The interpersonal stressor (whether to go out with her friends to eat) and the subsequent intense emotional upset while being alone combined to trigger the binge eating.

In terms of the behavioral features of BN, she was making steady progress towards establishing a regular pattern of eating. On all four days during the past week that she did not binge, she had succeeded in having at least something to eat for her meals and even managed to try some light snacks. Although she had a total of four binges and six episodes of purging this week (it is not unusual for some patients with severe BN to purge more frequently than they binge due to intense fears regarding weight gain), at the start of therapy she had been binge eating and purging nearly every day of the month and it was not unusual on weekends for her to purge several times.

TEXT BOX 4.4
Cognitive restructuring

Name: _____   Date: _____   Time: _____

SITUATION/TRIGGER Describe the event that led to the unpleasant feeling(s)	FEELINGS 1. Specify sad, anxious, etc. 2. Rate 1–100%	AUTOMATIC THOUGHTS What were you thinking? (Try not to censor your thoughts)	COGNITIVE DISTORTIONS (e.g., all-or-nothing, shoulds, etc.)	EVIDENCE FOR THOUGHTS	EVIDENCE AGAINST THOUGHTS
Asked my girlfriend to go away for the weekend with me She said she would like to but could not make it this weekend	Anxious (80%) Terrible ... don't know ... so upset, embarrassed, rejected (100%)	She doesn't want to come with me because I'm fat ... who could blame her, I can't stand looking at me either	Labeling Mind-reading others' thoughts or reasons		Girlfriend frequently travels with me Girlfriend has traveled with me and we've had fun even when I weighed more than now
Dinner		I should not eat ... I'm not going to eat now ... I'm going to skip dinner and go exercise ... it beats throwing up. I have to look better so that she will want to see me	Shoulds, Dichotomous (all-or-none thinking)		

RESTRUCTURED THOUGHTS or REASONED CONCLUSION *"Is there any other way of looking at this?"*

I feel fat but that doesn't mean I am fat. If I skip dinner and go exercise I'm just setting myself up to binge later. I have to keep going through this in my head. I really have no evidence that she didn't want to go away with me because I'm fat. I have to stop calling myself fat ... she never does and she gets upset with me when I do it. No, I just have to believe her that she couldn't go away this weekend. She usually says yes.

COMMENTS

Patients with BN, other forms of eating disorders, and other psychiatric problems (such as depression, anxiety, fears, etc.) tend to have certain maladaptive or problematic thoughts that serve to maintain the specific problem. In the case of eating disorders, patients typically have maladaptive thoughts about their eating, weight, shape and these things influence their self-worth. Of course, other types of maladaptive thoughts that include self-esteem, self-worth, or trigger strong emotions such as anxiety, depression, or anger can also be present. The concept of cognitive restructuring, which is another hallmark or critical component of CBT, is that it is possible to identify, challenge, and change these types of maladaptive thoughts.

Although there are many types of maladaptive thoughts that such patients experience, there are certain types of thoughts that are especially common or typical. One particularly frequent theme or example of a maladaptive thoughts is "dichotomous thinking" (i.e., all-or-none or black-or-white thoughts such as food is either good or bad, a dieter is completely in control or is out of control). Another theme that is most salient to patients with eating disorders is the overevaluation of shape/weight (e.g., achieving thinness is essential for happiness or success, one cannot be loved if one is not thin).

The process of cognitive restructuring, like self-monitoring, requires a collaborative stance between the therapist and the patient. Cognitive restructuring builds upon the successes of the self-monitoring efforts and the increased self-awareness of patients. The first step is to increase self-awareness to try to identify thoughts as they occur. A critical concept is that many of the maladaptive thoughts have become "automatic" and are no longer questioned. An excellent example to demonstrate this concept to patients is to have them think about driving a manual transmission ("stick shift") car. Once a person becomes an experienced driver, it seems to occur naturally or automatically. It is easy to see, however, how many thoughts and decisions a driver must make on a regular basis (e.g., when to turn, how much to turn, when to shift up or down, when to press the clutch, what to do when braking so as not to stall the car, etc.). These many and ongoing thoughts have become "automatic" for a driver. The first critical lesson is that even though the thoughts are automatic (not completely consciously aware of) they clearly influence behaviors. Continuing with the example of driving, inquire what typically happens to a driver when they almost encounter an accident or pass a police officer while going too fast. These typical events tend to make the person a bit more "aware" of their "automatic" thinking about driving. The second critical lesson is that it is possible to become increasingly aware of one's thinking and its relationship to behaviors and choices. Returning to the example of driving, if a driver from the United States wishes to drive effectively in the United Kingdom, it is necessary to change the automatic thoughts about driving to allow safe driving on the different side of the road. The third lesson is that it is possible to modify or change such automatic thoughts if it is indicated.

Steps for cognitive restructuring

A variety of cognitive restructuring forms are available in the CBT manuals referenced throughout this text. Above is a modified example of a cognitive restructuring form used at Yale. Once the rationale is explained to patients, they are encouraged to follow the following steps. This process requires practice and is enhanced by feedback from the therapist on a regular basis. Cognitive restructuring is a major component of the second phase of CBT for BN (Fairburn, Marcus, & Wilson, 1993b).

Step 1 involves identifying and specifically noting problematic thoughts during specific situations (e.g., during decisions to skip meals, before binge eating, during upsetting situations, etc.). Step 2 involves treating the thought as a hypothesis or possibility and trying to determine the validity or accuracy of the thought. In essence, the patient needs to weigh evidence for and against the thought in order to challenge it. Step 3 involves either restructuring (changing the thought) or arriving at a different possible way of thinking about the situation (a "reasoned conclusion").

Future directions

Improving treatments

Even among CBT studies that have produced the most impressive outcomes, a substantial proportion of patients do not recover. It is therefore important (a) to find ways to predict who will respond adequately to treatments; and (b) to find ways to improve treatments. Finding reliable predictors of treatment outcomes for BN has proven to be difficult (Reas, Schoemaker, Zipfel, & Williamson, 2001; Reas, Williamson, Martin, & Zucker, 2000; Wilson, 2005; Wilson et al., 1999). In contrast to the difficulty in identifying patient predictors of outcome, studies of BN have identified rapid early response to treatment as a significant predictor of positive treatment outcome (Agras et al., 2000a; Fairburn, Agras, Walsh, Wilson, & Stice, 2004b; Wilson et al., 1999, 2002). For example, Fairburn et al. (2004) found that the treatment responders in the Agras et al. (2000a) study had a mean 59% change (in purging) from baseline to the fourth week. This raises the possibility that non-responders (or slow responders) can be quickly identified who might benefit from additional or alternative treatment. Potential examples of this approach could be to try alternative treatments, different medications, or motivational methods with the non-responders.

Another important avenue for research is to investigate how different treatments might achieve their outcomes. Research with BN has progressed sufficiently to the point where efficacious treatments have been found and treatment studies have become larger and more sophisticated. Research is beginning to explore potential ways in which treatments work (Wilson et al., 1999, 2002) and complementing this research with naturalistic longitudinal studies (Fairburn, Stice, Cooper, Doll, Normanm & O'Connor, 2003b).

Dissemination

The majority of patients with BN who seek additional treatment at specialized eating disorder centers do not appear to have received empirically supported treatments in the past. For example, Crow, Mussel, Peterson, Knopke, and Mitchell (1999) found that 96.5% of a group of BN patients had received some form of psychotherapy, but only 6.9% reported having received CBT. Of those with prior treatment, 63.7% had been prescribed various medications, with fluoxetine being the most common. Of those respondents who were given fluoxetine, only 36.6% reported having been prescribed a dose of at least 60 mg/day, which is the established dosage for BN (FBNCSG, 1992). Thus, many patients with BN treated in general practice settings appear to receive inadequate pharmacotherapy (insufficient dosing and/or inadequate duration) or unspecified psychotherapies lacking empirical support. Unfortunately, this is a problem that is not unique to eating disorders. There is clear evidence that interventions found to be effective for a variety of other behavior and health concerns are not being disseminated into widespread clinical practice (Glasgow, Lichtenstein, & Marcus, 2003; McGlynn et al., 2003).

Research on the treatment of BN has provided impressive support for certain treatments. CBT has been found to have "efficacy" in carefully conducted and controlled studies in specialized centers and appears to have "effectiveness" in emerging research with non-specialists in diverse clinical settings. The next challenge is to achieve broader dissemination. In the UK there has been an aggressive national public health movement towards requiring clinicians to select and provide those treatments that have been established based on research (NICE, 2004). The impact of such governmental and policy actions will naturally be examined over time. In terms of future research on treatment, the importance of dissemination is becoming the focus of greater interest. For example, new frameworks and approaches to plan and design studies of health behavior change have been developed (Glasgow, Klesges, Dzewaltowski, Bull, & Estabrooks, 2004; Klesges, Estabrooks, Dzewaltowski, Bull, & Glasgow, 2005).

Summary

Bulimia nervosa is characterized by recurrent binge eating, regular use of inappropriate weight control methods (most frequently self-induced vomiting), severe dietary restraint, and the overevaluation of weight and shape. BN is a serious psychiatric disorder and is associated with increased risk for a number of medical and psychosocial problems. Since most persons with BN are average weight and many are secretive and embarrassed about the problem, many cases go unnoticed and untreated. This is unfortunate since it appears to be a relatively chronic problem if untreated and it causes those afflicted with it considerable distress and unhappiness. A number of effective treatments have been identified, most notably a specific form of psychotherapy (CBT) and – to a lesser extent – antidepressant medications. In addition, research has found that CBT may be effective for some patients even with minimal therapist involvement. Pressing needs for further research include developing treatments for those patients who fail to improve with existing interventions and finding ways to translate and disseminate effective treatments into mainstream clinical practice.

Atypical eating disorders and binge eating disorder 5
Assessment and treatment

Introduction

The atypical eating disorders (eating disorder not otherwise specified, EDNOS) are the most common eating disorders but also the least studied. One specific example of EDNOS is binge eating disorder (BED), which is also included in the DSM-IV as a research category. As summarized in chapter 2, the various forms of atypical eating disorders labeled EDNOS are distributed across age and weight categories in complex and poorly understood ways. The few available clinical studies suggest that persons with EDNOS have problems that resemble those seen in anorexia nervosa and bulimia nervosa, except perhaps at different symptom levels or in different combinations (Fairburn & Harrison, 2003). This may be especially true for adolescents (Eating Disorders Commission, 2005). BED is associated with older age and with substantially increased risk of obesity and therefore the various medical issues associated with obesity (chapter 6). It seems that a core feature which cuts across these various categories of eating problems is the overevaluation of shape and weight. This feature seems present, to varying degrees, in most cases. With that context in mind, this chapter begins with an overview of the major assessment issues relevant to EDNOS and BED. The major research findings about treatments will then be summarized.

Assessment of atypical eating disorders and binge eating disorder

The main assessment issues reviewed for anorexia nervosa (chapter 3) and for bulimia nervosa (chapter 4) are relevant for EDNOS. Recent reviews of clinical and research observations of EDNOS concluded that most forms of these atypical eating disorders appear to resemble anorexia nervosa and bulimia nervosa except for the severity levels or combinations of symptoms (Fairburn & Bohn, in press; Fairburn & Harrison, 2003). Thus, the behavioral, psychological, and medical issues reviewed for anorexia nervosa and bulimia nervosa are relevant here. Clinically, it is worth emphasizing the importance of broad assessment rather than over-reliance on just a few "typical" features such as amenorrhea, binge eating, or vomiting. For example, general questions asking about body image may reveal significant distress in a person who denies (or prefers to remain secretive about) any concerns about weight or eating. Another example is to ask about laxative, diet, and diuretic misuse, rather than just focusing on self-induced vomiting. Finally, asking about exercise might be a "safer" topic for certain patients who are strictly regulating their weight. In closing, it is worth reiterating the high levels of shame and embarrassment that are characteristic of patients with bulimia-like presentations and the high level of denial that is especially characteristic of those with anorexia-like features.

Assessment instruments and atypical eating disorders

Research with some of the major questionnaires and interview instruments has generally supported their use for detecting and assessing atypical eating disorders. These instruments have utility for screening in community studies (Mond et al., 2004) and for assessing patients across diverse age groups (Binford et al., 2004; Tanofsky-Kraff, Morgan, Yanovski, Marmarosh, Wilfley, & Yanovski, 2003), gender (Johnson, Kirk, & Reed, 2001), ethnicity (Grilo, Lozano, & Masheb, 2005), and different weight groups including obese (Celio, Wilfley, Crow, Mitchell, & Walsh, 2004; Grilo et al., 2001a, 2003b, 2004a; Reas et al., 2006) and extremely obese (Elder, Grilo, Masheb, Rothschild, Burke-Martindale, & Brody, 2006; Kalarchian, Wilson, Brolin, & Bradley, 2000) patients. The utility of these assessment methods does vary from instrument to instrument and they appear to perform slightly differently across different patient groups and settings (Gladis et al., 1998a). The variability in the performance of these measures for assessing atypical eating disorders does not seem to represent a departure from their usefulness for either bulimia nervosa (Keel, Crow, Davis, & Mitchell, 2002) or anorexia nervosa (Passi et al., 2003). In general, self-report methods are less useful for younger groups and for distinguishing more ambiguous types of symptoms (undereating or overeating). Another general finding is that self-report measures yield higher levels of concerns about eating, weight, and shape than interview methods. The reader is referred to recent comprehensive reviews of these various assessment issues (Grilo, 2005; Mitchell & Peterson, 2005).

Medical assessment and co-morbidities

As noted above, the medical assessments and issues should roughly parallel the detailed review provided for anorexia nervosa (chapter 3), bulimia nervosa (chapter 4), and obesity (chapter 6) depending on the nature of the prominent symptoms present in EDNOS. In particular, BED is associated with increased BMI and obesity (Spitzer et al., 1992; Telch, Agras, & Rossiter, 1988; Wilfley et al., 2003) and may represent a risk factor for subsequent or further weight gain (Agras et al., 1997). Thus, the obesity-related assessments in chapter 6 are especially relevant for BED. In addition, however, this chapter will call special attention to the need for assessing potential diabetes-related problems. The focus in this chapter will be on the association between certain forms of disordered eating and diabetes. Chapter 6 will discuss type II diabetes as a major health problem associated with obesity.

Atypical eating disorders and diabetes

Approximately 30 published studies have examined the frequency of disordered eating behaviors and clinical eating disorders in patients with type I insulin dependent diabetes (IDDM) and with type II non-insulin dependent diabetes (NIDDM) (e.g., Crow, Kendall, Praus, & Thuras 2001; Herpertz et al., 1998; see review by Herpertz & Nielsen, 2003). The majority of research has focused on IDDM. See Text Box 5.1 for a description of different types of diabetes.

Overall, anorexia nervosa does not co-occur at an elevated rate with type I or IDDM, but problems with binge eating (bulimia nervosa, binge eating disorder, and EDNOS) are found at rates two to three times higher than expected (Crow et al., 2001; Herpertz & Nielsen, 2003; Mannucci, Rotella, Ricca, Moretti, Placidi, & Rotella, 2005). See Table 5.1 for a model for understanding the co-occurrence

TEXT BOX 5.1

Diabetes

Diabetes is a serious medical problem (a "metabolic" disorder). It refers to problems in which the body does not produce insulin or properly use insulin. Insulin, a hormone, is needed by the body to convert glucose (sugar) into energy. The exact or specific causes of diabetes remains uncertain but it is well established that obesity, unhealthy eating, and insufficient physical activity play important roles in the development and maintenance of diabetes. Current estimates are that over 18 million people (6.3%) in the United States have diabetes (American Diabetes Association; www.diabtes.org).

MAJOR TYPES OF DIABETES

There are three major types of diabetes (type I, type II, and gestational diabetes). Interested readers can consult two publications available from the American Diabetes Association that contain practical information about diagnosis, treatment, and lifestyle management guidelines based on scientifically rigorous and updated information (*Diabetes: A Guide to Living Well; and A Field Guide to Type 2 Diabetes*).

Type I diabetes refers to insulin dependent diabetes (IDDM). IDDM results from the body's inability to produce insulin (the pancreas does not secrete enough insulin) and this deficiency prevents glucose from being converted into energy. Treatment of IDDM is complex. It involves close monitoring of blood sugar levels, multiple daily insulin injections, and very careful restriction of eating (specific times and specific foods) to help maintain reasonably normal blood sugar levels. Medical complications are frequent and serious (they affect all organ systems including the kidneys, retina, cardiovascular) when metabolic control is poor. Approximately 5% to 10% of diabetes cases are type I.

Type II diabetes refers to non-insulin dependent diabetes (NIDDM). NIDDM results from insulin resistance which refers to the body's failure to use insulin properly (energy producing cells ignore the insulin). In many cases, weight loss, healthy and balanced eating, and increased physical activity can improve NIDDM and decrease the necessity for or the amount of medication. Approximxately 90% of diabetes cases in the United States are type II.

Gestational diabetes refers to a form of diabetes that affects approximately 4% of pregnant women.

Pre-diabetes refers to a condition that is defined as higher than normal blood glucose levels but not high enough for the diagnosis of type II diabetes. "Pre-diabetes" has been found to frequently progress to diabetes and is therefore a signal to intervene preventatively before a more serious problem develops. The American Diabetes Association has estimated that over 40 million people in the United States have pre-diabetes (in addition to the over 18 million with diabetes).

Diagnosis

Assessment of diabetes is critical for management and is relatively straightforward. Unfortunately, many persons do not obtain these tests and the American Diabetes Association has

continues

estimated that over 5 million people (approximately 30%) in the United States with diabetes are unaware that they have the problem.

To assess for diabetes, two tests can be used: the Fasting Plasma Glucose Test (FPG) or an Oral Glucose Tolerance Test (OGTT). The FPG is used more frequently because it is easier, faster, and less costly. Frequently, to confirm the diagnosis, a health professional may repeat the test or administer the second test. With the FPG, a fasting blood glucose level of 126 mg/dl or higher signals the presence of diabetes; a level between 100 and 125 reflects "pre-diabetes." With the OGTT (a test in which the person's blood glucose level is measured after fasting and performed two hours after taking a glucose-rich drink), a level above 200 mg/dl reflects diabetes and a level between 140 mg/dl and 199 mg/dl reflects "pre-diabetes."

of eating disorders and diabetes. An important issue concerns the potential misuse or omission of insulin as an inappropriate method for weight control.

Less research has focused on eating disorders in persons with type II or NIDDM. That body of research has consistently found elevated rates of binge eating (Herpertz & Nielsen, 2003; Kenardy et al., 1994, 2001). Kenardy, Mensch, Bowen, and Pearson (1994) reported that 14% of newly diagnosed NIDDM cases reported binge eating at least twice weekly, a significantly higher frequency than the 4% rate among an age- and BMI-matched control group. More recent studies of NIDDM patients have reported rates of BED generally ranging 21% to 35% (Crow, Keel, & Kendall, 1998; Kenardy, Mensch, Bowen, Green, Walton, & Dalton, 2001), which is substantially higher than the rate of BED found in the general population (Striegel-Moore & Franko, 2003). See Table 5.1 for a model for understanding the co-occurrence of eating disorders and diabetes. An important issue concerns the potential misuse or omission of insulin as an inappropriate method for weight control.

An important finding is that most type II diabetic patients who are binge eaters report that they started binge eating many years before their diabetes developed (Herpertz et al., 1998; Herpertz & Nielsen, 2003). Thus, binge eating may represents a risk for developing type II diabetes and does not result from dieting attempts to cope with diabetes, a conclusion also voiced by the NFT (2000a) for non-diabetics. In addition, since binge eating also increases the risk for continued weight gain (NFT, 2000b; Yanovski, 2003) this may increase the risk for "pre-diabetes" or the progression to type II NIDDM. In chapter 6, it will be noted that the prevalence of NIDDM in the United States is increasing substantially and in a manner that parallels the increased prevalence of obesity.

TABLE 5.1

Model of co-occurrence of eating disorder psychopathology and diabetes

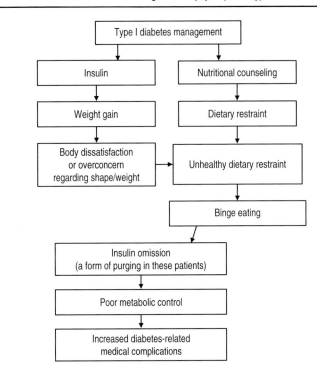

COMMENT

The above schematic diagram provides a useful model for thinking about the co-occurrence of eating disorder psychopathology and type I diabetes. Elevated rates of binge eating problems (bulimia nervosa, binge eating disorder, and atypical eating disorders classified as EDNOS) are found in patients with IDDM. In such cases, the required insulin therapy to address the IDDM produces weight gain and in some patients this results in overconcern regarding shape/weight which leads to unhealthy dietary restraint. In turn, unhealthy restraint may trigger binge eating, which in turn results in both weight gain and intensified concerns about the weight gain. This leads some patients to omit insulin when they believe that they have overeaten or binged. In such cases, the insulin omission can be thought of as an inappropriate weight compensatory behavior akin to purging behaviors in bulimia nervosa. Although anorexia nervosa does not occur at elevated rates in patients with IDDM, if it does occur great care needs to be taken to determine whether they are omitting insulin as an additional method to sustain their abnormally low weight. Insulin omission is serious, results in poor metabolic control, and can hasten the development of serious diabetes-related medical complications.

Assessment of non-medical factors

Psychological factors

BED is often associated with a broad range of psychological distress and co-existing psychiatric problems, including depression, anxiety disorders, and personality disorders (Bulik, Sullivan, & Kendler, 2002; Grilo et al., 2001a; Marcus, Wing, Ewing, Kern, McDermott, & Gooding, 1990; Schwalberg et al., 1992; Spitzer et al., 1992; Wilfley et al., 2000; Yanovski, Nelson, Dubbert, & Spitzer, 1993). The rates for many of these co-occurring psychiatric problems are comparable to those observed in other psychiatric patient groups (Wilfley et al., 2000) and are higher than observed in non-psychiatric comparison groups of obese patients who do not binge eat (Yanovski et al., 1993). Grilo and colleagues (2003b) reported that adult patients with EDNOS did not differ significantly from patients with bulimia nervosa in the co-occurrence of personality disorders.

Typically, in treatment-seeking patients with BED, studies generally find that roughly 50% have mood disorders (most commonly major depressive disorder), 35% have at least one anxiety disorder, and roughly 20% have an alcohol or drug use disorder (Grilo, Masheb, & Wilson, 2005c; White & Grilo, 2006; Wilfley et al., 2002). Grilo and colleagues (2001a) found that patients who were classified as negative affect dietary types (Stice & Agras, 1999) – based on higher levels of depressive affect alongside lower self-esteem – had significantly higher rates of major depressive disorder and dythymia than pure dietary subtypes. High levels of body image dissatisfaction are common in BED patients and comparable to levels seen in patients with BN (Barry et al., 2003). These findings highlight the complexity of these patients and indicate the need for thorough psychiatric evaluations.

Eating behaviors and nutrition

Studies have also found that persons with BED differ from obese non-bingers on most dieting and weight history variables (Allison et al., 2005; Brody, Walsh, & Devlin, 1994; Marcus, Wing, & Hopkins, 1988; Spitzer et al., 1992, 1993). In general, obese patients with BED have more chaotic eating patterns and histories of greater weight variability or weight cycling than obese non-bingers. Aside from the binge eating episodes, obese patients with BED report eating significantly more meals during the week, having more episodes of overeating than obese patients (Allison et al., 2005) and frequently report overeating in response to various emotional states (Masheb & Grilo, 2006). In addition to these chaotic eating patterns during the day, obese patients with BED report night eating significantly more frequently than obese non-bingers (Allison et al., 2005). Grilo and Masheb (2004) reported that roughly 25% of obese patients with BED had night eating episodes with roughly 9% having night eating on at least half of the nights each month. BED patients with night eating problems tended to be heavier. These findings suggest that different forms of disordered eating can combine to contribute to obesity (Tanofsky-Kraff & Yanovski, 2004).

The clinical observations regarding the chaotic quality and extent of overeating and binge eating behaviors in BED have been supported by a variety of laboratory studies (Walsh & Boudreau, 2003). Obese binge eaters, for example, are generally able to consume more food than obese non-bingers when instructed to overeat in laboratory settings (Guss et al., 2002; Yanovski et al., 1992). Collectively, these findings highlight the complexity of these patients relative to their obese peers. Research has supported the utility of some of the main eating disorder assessment methods as reviewed earlier for AN and BN. In particular, the self-report inventories, the Questionnaire on Eating Patterns (Yanovski, 1993) and the Eating Disorder Examination – Questionnaire version (Fairburn & Beglin, 1994) have received empirical support for their utility with these diverse eating disorder patients (Elder et al., 2006; Grilo et al., 2001a, 2001b; Reas et al., 2006).

The challenges in establishing healthy and normalized eating described in chapter 6 are undoubtedly relevant for BED. Unfortunately, at the present time relatively little is known about either the nature of these disturbances or the best ways to intervene clinically. This dearth of knowledge has led experts to emphasize the need for research to precisely characterize the behavioral and metabolic nature of various forms of disordered eating and eating disorders (Tanofsky-Kraff & Yanovski, 2004; Yanovski, 2003).

Treatments for atypical eating disorders

Treatment needs

Almost no research exists on treatment for patients with atypical eating disorders or EDNOS, except for the specific subgroup diagnosed as having BED. Treatment research on BED will be described later. Clinical studies suggest that persons with EDNOS have problems that resemble those seen in anorexia nervosa and bulimia nervosa except for the levels or combinations of some criteria. This may be especially true for adolescents (Eating Disorders Commission, 2005). The three available studies of natural course and outcome suggest that EDNOS has a fairly persistent course over time, although there seems to be considerable variation in the nature of the symptoms (Grilo et al., 2003b; Herzog et al., 1993; Milos, Spindler, Schnyder, & Fairburn, 2005). These clinical data highlight the need for research on how best to treat these common eating problems currently labeled as EDNOS.

Pharmacotherapy

There appears to be only one published controlled treatment study with a clearly defined patient group that would fit the diagnosis of EDNOS. McCann and Agras (1990) reported that desipramine (an antidepressant) was significantly superior to placebo for reducing binge eating in a patient group described as having "non-purging bulimia nervosa." This study is consistently incorrectly cited in the literature as an early study of BED. This is because the term "non-purging bulimia" was widely used in the late 1980s and early 1990s until the term BED was adopted along with the final research criteria (Spitzer et al., 1992, 1993). Indeed, two of the first controlled studies of psychotherapy for BED referred to these patients as having non-purging bulimia (Telch, Agras, Rossiter, Wilfley, & Kenardy, 1990; Wilfley et al., 1993). Unlike the psychotherapy studies, however, the patients in the McCann and Agras (1990) pharmacotherapy study were severely restricting their food intake in between their episodes of binge eating. Although they did not use self-induced vomiting, their extreme food restriction suggests that they were more accurately EDNOS or perhaps BN restricting type, but certainly not BED. These diagnostic issues and complexities notwithstanding, this study essentially found that an antidepressant with efficacy for bulimia nervosa produced similar outcomes in EDNOS. Interestingly, and unfortunately, the patients in the McCann and Agras (1990) study relapsed within four weeks of discontinuing the medication.

Current guidelines and future treatment directions

The NICE (2004) treatment guidelines include the common sense advice: "In the absence of evidence to guide the management of eating disorders not otherwise specified, other than binge eating disorder, it is recommended that the clinician considers following the guidance on the treatment of the eating problem that most closely resembles the individual patient's eating disorder"(p. 71). Thus, the clinician can follow and apply the treatments or treatment components that seem most aligned with the patient's clinical presentation. This basic advice has been echoed by leading experts in their recent treatment reviews (Fairburn & Harrison, 2003; Wilson, 2005; Wilson & Shafran, 2005). Recently, Fairburn, Cooper, and Shafran (2003a) have described a "transdiagnostic model" for assessment and treatment. This model focuses on factors or mechanisms that may maintain different forms of eating disorders (rather than focusing on diagnosis) and suggests interventions tailored to those specific needs. This model suggests that instead of relying on current categories of diagnoses that clinicians should focus on specifically identifying eating disorder symptoms that are present along with additional psychological needs (e.g., highly perfectionistic thinking; low self-esteem, interpersonal deficits) or temperamental factors (e.g., negative or depressive affect, impulsivity, etc.) that need to be specifically targeted. This "new model" or approach builds on the past decade of advances in CBT for eating disorders and makes use of our increased knowledge. Research is ongoing at Oxford University testing this approach.

Some of the basic concepts in this new "transdiagnostic model" (Fairburn et al., 2003a) have longstanding traditions in the behavior therapy field. In an early example, Loro and Orleans (1981) provided recommendations regarding how behavioral and functional analyses of binge eating could guide treatment. More recently, a well-articulated treatment approach can be found in the Therapeutic Contract Program (TCP) developed by Levendusky (Berglas & Levendusky, 1985; Heinssen, Levendusky, & Hunter, 1995; Levendusky, Willis, & Ghinassi, 1994).

The TCP (Levendusky et al., 1994) emphasizes individualized assessment of patients' symptoms and needs in relation to psychosocial strengths and deficits. The TCP involves the patient "as colleague" in the collaborative treatment process (Heinssen et al., 1995). The first step involves identifying and prioritizing immediate problems (both eating disorder specific and broader psychosocial functioning context). This assessment is then used to establish short and intermediate term goals. Specific interventions that are most suited to the specific problems and goals are used. This method de-emphasizes the importance of "diagnosis," and instead focuses on person-specific problems. The TCP then provides guidance in how to select research-supported interventions to address the specific problems (Heinssen et al., 1995). One study reported, based on a non-randomized, non-controlled comparison, that a group of patients with severe but diverse forms of eating disorders derived greater benefit from TCP than from traditional inpatient hospitalization (Levendusky et al., 1994).

Overview of treatments for binge eating disorder

History

Yanovski (1993), in the first comprehensive review of emerging research in this area, evaluated treatment studies with broad categories of obese patients, many with binge eating problems. Following reports that obese binge eaters frequently experienced difficulties with weight loss programs (Marcus et al., 1988), one approach was to compare the treatment responses of obese binge eaters and non-binge eaters to various types of obesity treatments (see chapter 6). Although not unequivocal (e.g., Wadden, Foster, & Letizia, 1992), many of the first-generation treatment studies reported that obese binge eaters benefited less from diverse weight loss programs than did obese patients who did not binge eat (e.g., Marcus et al., 1988; Yanovski, Gormally, Leser, Gwirtsman, & Yanovski, 1994). These concerns were consistent with some clinical views at the time that dieting exacerbated binge eating in binge eaters in the same manner that restrictive dieting plays a potent role in the maintenance of bulimia nervosa. These initial concerns led to some researchers adapting and testing psychological and pharmacological treatments that had been well established for bulimia nervosa in patients with BED.

Dieting and BED

A thorough and balanced review of the body of research pertaining to this issue concluded that concerns that dieting induces eating or psychological disorders in overweight adults are not supported by research (NFT, 2000b). A recent randomized controlled intervention study designed specifically to test this issue found that two different types of diets (a highly restrictive liquid meal replacement diet and a moderate balanced deficit diet) did not result in greater binge eating or psychological distress than a non-diet condition (Wadden et al., 2004). More recent treatment research (Gladis, Wadden, Vogt, Foster, Kuehnel, & Bartlett, 1998b; Sherwood, Jeffery, & Wing, 1998) has reopened the debate about the potential role of obesity treatments in BED.

Treatment needs

Research on the treatment of BED is still in its early stages. The inclusion of this research category in the diagnostic system (DSM-IV) appears to have facilitated or encouraged increased research attention (Grilo et al., 1997). For considering treatment research, it is important to keep in mind that patients with BED suffer from problems in four domains (Grilo et al., 2001a; Wilfley et al., 2003): (1) binge eating; (2) attitudinal features of eating disorders; (3) psychological symptoms and distress; (4) obesity, along with its associated health risks and, if present, medical problems. Thus, treatments need to be able to address all of these problem areas (Goldfein, Devlin, & Spitzer, 2000). Overall, research on the treatment of BED can be summarized as follows. CBT is widely considered to be the best available treatment for persons with BED (NICE, 2004), although it does not appear to produce weight loss. There is also some support for other psychological, behavioral, and pharmacological approaches, although this is based on fewer studies. Although BED is the most researched form of the atypical eating disorders, there are considerably fewer well-controlled treatment studies than for bulimia nervosa reviewed in chapter 4. A review of the major approaches and findings follows.

Pharmacotherapy

Pharmacotherapy versus placebo for BED has been compared in several randomized placebo-controlled studies (Alger, Schwalberg, Bigaouette, Michalek, & Howard, 1991; Appolinario et al., 2003; Arnold, McElroy, Hudson, Welge, Bennett, & Keck, 2002; Grilo, Masheb, & Wilson, 2005c; Hudson et al., 1998; McCann & Agras, 1990; McElroy et al., 2000; McElroy et al., 2003a, 2003b; Stunkard, Berkowitz, Tanrikut, Reiss, & Young, 1996a). Most of these studies tested antidepressant medications. Of the remaining studies, two

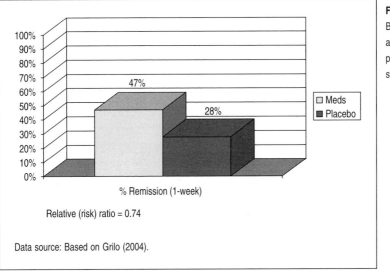

Figure 5.1.
Binge eating
abstinence rates in
pharmacotherapy
studies for BED.

tested obesity medications (Appolinario et al., 2003; Stunkard et al., 1996a) and one tested an antiepileptic medication (McElroy et al., 2003a). Overall, most pharmacotherapy studies have been of short duration (< 12 weeks, except for 16 weeks in Grilo et al. (2005c) and have yet to report follow-up data (except for Stunkard et al., 1996a). Most of the pharmacotherapy studies have focused on binge eating and weight and have given little attention to the effects on eating disorder psychopathology. Overall, attrition rates in pharmacotherapy trials have ranged 14% to 54% with an average of about 35%.

Most, but not all, controlled pharmacotherapy studies for BED (Alger et al., 1991; Grilo et al., 2005c), reported significantly greater reductions in binge eating for medications than for placebo. Figure 5.1 provides a summary of a meta-analysis recently performed by Grilo (2004) on outcomes from controlled studies for BED. Overall, across studies, pharmacotherapy resulted in a higher rate of remission (one week) from binge eating than did placebo (47% versus 28%, respectively). The statistically significant differences observed for pharmacotherapy relative to placebo for BED are not particularly robust from a clinical perspective (Grilo, 2004; NICE, 2004). The meta-analysis completed by NICE (2004) and the recent meta-analysis performed by Grilo (2004), including several new studies not considered by NICE (2004), both concluded, based on effect-size measures of clinical significance that there is insufficient evidence to support pharmacotherapy for BED. Lastly, the only

Figure 5.2.
Binge eating
abstinence rates for
different classes of
medication.

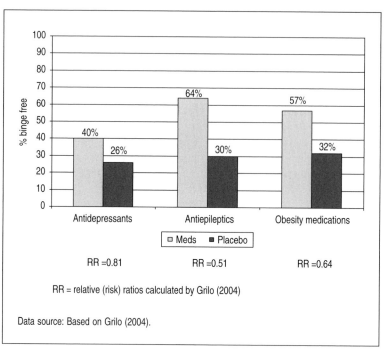

available published follow-up data for pharmacotherapy-only treatment suggests that relapse occurs rapidly (within one to four months) after discontinuing the medication (Stunkard, Berkowitz, Tanrikut, Reiss, & Young, 1996a).

Figure 5.2 summarizes the findings from the meta-analysis by Grilo (2004) separately for the different classes (antidepressants, antiepileptic, and obesity medications). Overall, there does not appear to be substantial difference in the efficacy of the different medications tested for BED relative to placebo. The largest clinical effect comes from the one study with an antiepileptic (topiramate). McElroy et al. (2003a), in a 14-week randomized double-blind trial with 61 obese BED patients, reported that topiramate resulted in a remission rate (no binges during fourteenth week endpoint) of 64% versus 30% for placebo. Translating this finding into an estimate of clinical effect (RR = relative risk), topiramate resulted in a 50% increase in the likelihood of a one-week remission. Topiramate is associated with numerous side effects and this medication resulted in a 47% attrition rate during this trial. A more recent open-label longer term study of topiramate reported that roughly 70% of BED patients discontinued this medication (McElroy et al., 2004).

What about weight loss?

Several pharmacotherapy studies have reported statistically significant weight loss (Appolarino et al., 2003; Hudson et al., 1998; McElroy et al., 2000, 2003a, 2003b). Only two of these studies (Appolarino et al., 2003; McElroy et al., 2003a), however, found weight losses that were close to being clinically meaningful (7.4 kg, 5.9 kg, respectively). As noted above, the one study with topiramate (McElroy et al., 2003a) has very high attrition because of problems with side effects. The other medication showing some potential for producing weight loss in this patient group is sibutramine (Appolarino et al., 2003). In this study with 60 obese patients with BED, those receiving sibutramine lost an average of 7.4 kg, while those receiving placebo gained an average 1.4 kg. In this study, sibutramine had a low dropout rate (20%) and had a higher remission rate from binge eating than placebo (52% versus 32%). Sibutramine is an FDA-approved medication for obesity, where it has been the focus of a large number of studies with many patients (reviewed later in chapter 6).

Cognitive behavioral therapy (CBT) and psychological approaches for BED

Different forms of cognitive behavioral therapy (CBT) for BED have been compared to other treatment conditions including wait-list controls, behavioral weight loss treatments, and alternative methods of psychotherapy (Agras et al., 1994; Grilo & Masheb, 2005; Nauta, Hospers, Gerjo, & Jansen, 2000; Peterson, Mitchell, Engbloom, Nugent, Mussell, & Miller, 1998; Porzelius et al., 1995; Telch et al., 1990; Wilfley et al., 1993, 2002). Overall, the attrition rates for CBT across these studies range 10% to 35% (average of roughly 20%), which is lower than those found in the briefer pharmacotherapy studies.

CBT, which generally produces roughly 50% remission rates from binge eating, has consistently been found to be significantly superior to wait-list controls. An alternative form of CBT, known as dialectical behavior therapy (DBT), which focuses on emotion regulation and coping skills, has also been found to have efficacy (Telch, Agras, & Linehan, 2001). Two studies (Wilfley et al., 1993, 2002) reported that CBT and interpersonal psychotherapy (IPT) did not differ from each other but both produced significant and clinically impressive improvements in binge eating, with remission rates of 79% and 73%, respectively. Both of these treatments produced substantial improvements in eating disorder psychopathology and psychological well-being that were very well maintained for 12 months after finishing treatments. Other studies have also reported that the improvements achieved with various forms of CBT are well maintained (Carter & Fairburn, 1998; Peterson et al., 2001). See Text Box 5.2 for a sample of a self-monitoring and food record of a patient with BED receiving CBT. It is instructive to compare and contrast the eating patterns with those recorded by a patient with bulimia nervosa in the previous chapter (Text Box 4.3).

What about weight loss?

Despite these impressive reductions in binge eating, neither CBT nor IPT treatment resulted in significant weight loss. It is worth noting, however, that patients who achieved abstinence from binge eating did lose significantly more weight than those who did not stop binge eating. Such findings, also reported in other treatment studies (e.g., Grilo et al., 2005b), suggest that these interventions might at least prevent further weight gain (Yanovski, 2003) that is typically observed in untreated persons with BED (Fairburn et al., 2000).

Given the association between BED and obesity, it is surprising that only a few studies have directly compared various adaptations of CBT to behavioral weight loss (BWL) in BED. Two studies performed direct comparisons (Nauta et al., 2000; Porzelius, Houston, Smith, Arfken, & Fisher, 1995) and one study tested the addition of the treatments sequentially (Agras et al., 1994). Porzelius et al. (1995) found that the obese BED patients achieved similar reductions in binge eating in the CBT and BWL treatments and, contrary to expectation, lost significantly more weight in the CBT than in the BWL. Nauta et al. (2000) found that cognitive therapy was superior for reducing unhealthy attitudes regarding weight and shape but that behavioral therapy resulted in greater short-term weight loss which was subsequently regained. Agras and colleagues (1994) compared CBT, BWL, and desipramine. After three months of treatment, the CBT produced significantly greater reductions in binge eating than the BWL (67% vs. 44%) but the BWL resulted in statistically significantly more weight loss than CBT (2.0 kg vs. 0.7 kg). The addition of the medication desipramine did not enhance the treatments. By six months, the treatments did not differ significantly from each other. These treatment studies have not provided clear answers regarding

TEXT BOX 5.2
Daily self-monitoring and food record

Name: _____   Date: _____

Time of day (Time eating began and ended)	Type and quantity of food (provide as much detail as possible)	M = Meal S = Snack B = Binge	Setting (location, activity and others present)	Purging (how? how many times?)	Thoughts/feelings comments	Pre-meal hunger 0 = no hunger 10 = starving
7:00 a.m.	Toasted bagel with egg, sausage, and cheese, coffee roll; large regular coffee	Breakfast	Dunkin Donuts Drive-thru			
12:00 p.m.	2 beef burritos; 1 bean burrito; chips; x-large soda	Lunch	Taco-Bell restaurant			
1:30 p.m.	4 chocolate chip cookies		Work lounge with co-workers			
6:15 p.m.	Chips, dip, pretzels, soda		Home (alone), watching T.V.			
6:25 p.m.	2-3 crackers with cheese; half bowl left-over baked macaroni					
7:00 p.m.	4 slices pizza (sausage), chips, 2 sodas	Dinner			Order pizza delivery	
8:30 p.m.	4 slices pizza, bowl left-over baked macaroni - finished it, 3-4 handfuls chips, half left-over sandwich	Binge			Couldn't stop eating	

continues overleaf

TEXT BOX 5.2
continued

COMMENTS

This is a sample of a completed self-monitoring record from a 42-year-old married male who performs data management work. He lives alone with his wife (this is his second marriage) who is away because of a business trip for two days. This self-monitoring and food record covers one day and was completed one day after his first therapy session the week after completing a comprehensive evaluation at a university clinic. He presented to this clinic in response to an advertisement in the local paper for a study of binge eating. He had struggled with his weight since his mid-twenties, had tried numerous weight loss programs over the years, and had managed to lose weight many times only to gain it back. He responded to the advertisement because he was concerned about his continued weight gain (although his weight cycled over time the net result was an overall significant gain) and wondered whether he was a binge eater.

He reported always feeling great and empowered when he lost weight but especially demoralized when he ended up gaining it back. He described his feelings of embarrassment around having to buy several new wardrobes when he regained weight because as he lost the weight he was happy to throw away what he referred to as "fat clothes." He described feeling self-conscious about his weight but acknowledged that his wife always seemed interested in him regardless of his weight. When asked more about this, he acknowledged discomfort about his weight and wished he could change it ("or else I wouldn't have spent half my life going on and off diets"). Such weight concerns, while important, were not viewed as a major factor in how he viewed or evaluated his self-worth.

The comprehensive evaluation revealed that he met criteria for binge eating disorder in addition to being obese. It was difficult to get a clear picture of his eating and especially his overeating behaviors. At first, he had difficulty with the concept of "loss of control" but it soon became evident to him and the therapist that he did, in fact, regularly experience two different forms of overeating. He frequently overate (large amounts of food, large portion sizes, having seconds) but there were many instances of overeating that were very different. During these, he described feeling a sense of being "on cruise control" and "not being able to stop." As he thought about these overeating episodes, he elaborated that they were most frequently while alone and seemed to have a chaotic quality. Unlike his regular overeating, these episodes "on cruise control" usually involved grabbing and eating whatever foods happened to be available.

Inspection of this patient's self-monitoring and food record reveals this pattern clearly. The patient (over)eats throughout the day (generally large portions of unhealthy meals at breakfast and lunch; unhealthy snack at work). During the evening, a pattern seen in many patients with BED is evident. The patient begins the evening by eating a few unhealthy items, waits a while and then eats some more while waiting for dinner. The patient then overeats at dinner. So far, the patient exhibited what some have labeled as "grazing" and then overate at dinner. Then, roughly an hour after finishing a large dinner, the patient resumed eating but this time "lost control" and ate a very large amount of available food. Thus, the eating pattern is one of low dietary restraint, too much and disorganized overeating throughout the day, and binge eating. This is sharply different from the typical eating pattern of patients with bulimia who alternate between over-control (strict dietary restraint) and binge eating.

More broadly, this male patient's presenting picture of BED is fairly typical. In addition to the long history of struggling with overweight, this BED patient has less dietary restraint than is characteristic of BN (Masheb & Grilo, 2000). He also suffers from body image dissatisfaction but his level of overevaluation of shape and weight are less intense than generally seen in women with BED (Barry, Grilo, & Masheb, 2002). This patient experienced some difficulty in identifying or articulating instances of loss of control and he needed help in learning to identify thoughts and feelings as well as other possible triggers for the binge eating episodes.

the important question of whether CBT or BWL is more beneficial. These studies, however, have suggested, in contrast to the position held by some obesity experts (Gladis et al., 1998b), that behavioral weight loss programs do not seem to routinely result in weight loss in this specific subgroup of obese patients. One study that compared two different behavioral weight control treatments also reported that neither resulted in any weight loss (Goodrick, Poston Kimball, Reeves, & Foreyt, 1998).

Self-help forms of cognitive behavioral therapy

Recent controlled treatment studies with BED, like the findings for bulimia nervosa (chapter 4), have supported the utility of specific self-help adaptations of CBT (Grilo, 2000). CBT, adapted for guided self-help (CBTgsh) and/or pure self-help (CBTsh), has been tested in four controlled studies (Carter & Fairburn, 1998; Grilo & Masheb, 2005; Loeb, Wilson, Gilbert, & Labouvie, 2000; Peterson et al., 1998). CBTgsh and CBTsh have consistently been superior to controls for reducing binge eating and improving features of eating disorders. Overall, the controlled studies with guided self-help forms of CBT have reported roughly 50% remission rates. The self-help CBT treatments, like therapist-led CBT, do not result in weight loss.

Grilo and Masheb (2005) performed a randomized controlled study to test the relative efficacy of CBT and behavioral weight loss treatment (BWL) for BED both administered using guided self-help (CBTgsh and BWLgsh, respectively). This study also included a third control condition that partly controlled for attention effects. The findings from this study, which enrolled 90 obese men and women with BED, are summarized in the left three columns of Figure 5.3. As can be seen from Figure 5.3, the CBTgsh resulted in significantly higher rates of remission (46%) than both the BWLgsh (18%) and control condition (13%) which did not differ significantly from each other. This study provides strong support for the specific effectiveness of this form of CBT. To provide a context for interpreting the magnitude of the observed remission rates achieved using guided self-help, column 4 in Figure 5.3 shows the remission rates achieved by CBT given in traditional individual therapy format by specialized clinicians. Those data are abstracted from a controlled treatment

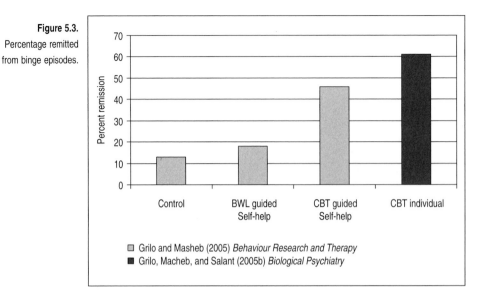

Figure 5.3.
Percentage remitted
from binge episodes.

Grilo and Masheb (2005) *Behaviour Research and Therapy*
Grilo, Macheb, and Salant (2005b) *Biological Psychiatry*

study performed by Grilo and colleagues (2005b) described later in this chapter. As is evident from Figure 5.3, the effects observed for CBTgsh are slightly lower than seen for CBT but they are certainly robust and superior to the BWLgsh and control treatments. Consistent with these findings, Peterson et al. (1998) found that guided self-help and therapist-led treatments using a modified form CBT were comparable.

Cognitive behavioral therapy and pharmacotherapy

To date, only one randomized placebo-controlled study has tested the efficacy of CBT and pharmacotherapy alone and in combination for BED (Grilo & Masheb, 2005). In this study, 108 patients with BED were randomized to one of four treatments for 16 weeks: fluoxetine, placebo, fluoxetine plus individual CBT, or placebo plus individual CBT. Attrition from the four different treatments was low (average 20%). CBT with placebo (61% remission) and CBT with fluoxetine (50% remission) did not significantly differ from each other but both were significant superior to fluoxetine (22% remission) and to placebo (26%) which did not differ from each other. Thus, CBT, but not fluoxetine, was found to be effective for BED. Weight loss, however, was modest and did not differ across treatments. Those patients who completely stopped binge eating, however, lost significantly more weight than those who did not.

The findings from the study by Grilo and Masheb (2005) are consistent with results from two other treatment studies that used different methods. Ricca and colleagues (2001), in a non-blinded study, found that CBT was more effective than fluoxetine alone and that the addition of fluoxetine to CBT did not improve the CBT outcomes. Devlin and colleagues (2005) found that adding fluoxetine did not improve behavioral weight loss outcomes more than placebo, whereas the addition of CBT significantly enhanced the outcomes. Collectively, these findings suggest that adding antidepressant medications to CBT or to BWL does not produce much added benefit. These recent findings echo the modest and inconsistent findings from the first generation of studies with obese binge eaters that combined medications with behavioral weight loss treatments (De Zwaan, Nutzinger, & Schoenbeck, 1992; Laederach-Hoffmann et al., 1999; Marcus et al., 1990).

A recent study tested the next logical clinical question. What about combining an obesity medication with CBT? Grilo, Masheb, and Salant (2005b) conducted a randomized placebo-controlled, double-blind study of an FDA-approved obesity medication (orlistat) given concurrently with guided self-help CBT (CBTgsh). Orlistat, is a noncentrally acting medication, with efficacy for weight loss in obese patients (reviewed in detail in chapter 6). Fifty obese patients with BED were provided CBTgsh and were, in addition, randomly assigned to 12-week treatments with either orlistat or placebo. Patients were followed in double-blind fashion for three months after completion and discontinuation of all treatments. Attrition was low (22%) and the medication was well tolerated. Figure 5.4 summarizes the two primary outcomes (remission from binge eating and achieving a 5% weight loss) determined at three months following treatment. As is evident from Figure 5.4, 52% of patients in both treatment conditions had remission from binge eating at the three-month follow-up. The addition of orlistat to CBTgsh resulted in a significantly greater proportion of patients with a 5% weight loss at three-month follow-up than did the addition of placebo to CBTgsh (32% versus 8%). Thus, the addition of orlistat to a form of CBT can facilitate weight loss in obese patients with BED. Overall, the clinical improvements were generally well maintained three months after treatment discontinuation.

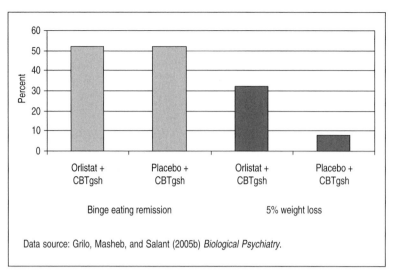

Figure 5.4.
Percentage of (n = 50) BED patients with remission from binge eating and 5% weight loss 3 months after treatments.

Data source: Grilo, Masheb, and Salant (2005b) *Biological Psychiatry*.

Future directions

Improving treatments

Finding ways to augment CBT, the best-established treatment for BED, to help facilitate weight loss in obese patients remains a pressing research need (Wilson & Fairburn, 2000). The addition of obesity medications to CBT, which received support in a recent study (Grilo et al., 2005b), might be a promising approach for clinicians and researchers to pursue. Treatment research on other forms of EDNOS and atypical eating disorders across the lifespan is also a high priority (Fairburn & Harrison, 2003; Wilson & Shafran, 2005).

Dissemination

Whether treatments found to work (efficacy) in specialized clinics can be effectively given in non-specialist primary care clinical settings is also uncertain. Obese persons with BED utilize high levels of health care (Johnson, Spitzer, & Williams, 2001; Striegel-Moore et al., 2004), but they are rarely given treatments that have been supported in specialized centers (Crow, Peterson, Levine, Thuras, & Mitchell, 2004; Striegel-Moore et al., 2004). There is some evidence that CBT by guided self-help can be effectively delivered by non-specialist clinicians in "real-world" clinical settings (Carter & Fairburn, 1998). Thus, it is important to find ways to disseminate these treatment approaches more broadly to diverse treatment settings. This has become, for example, a major national health care priority in the United Kingdom and the focus of aggressive ongoing efforts (NICE, 2004; Wilson & Shafran, 2005).

Summary

The atypical eating disorders – classified as EDNOS – are probably the most common forms of eating disorders but are the least studied. Available research on EDNOS suggests that these eating-related problems are not merely less severe forms or "subthreshold" to the other "formal" eating disorder categories. Recent years have seen considerable interest and research on BED, which is defined as regular binge eating without co-occurring extreme weight control methods. This interest is perhaps motivated clinically by the virtue of the significant association between binge eating and obesity. Indeed, BED has served as a useful bridge for dialogue between researchers in the fields of obesity and eating disorders. BED, in addition to its association with obesity and therefore heightened risk for medical problems, is associated with increased risk for psychosocial problems. Research has identified CBT as the best-established treatment for BED and recent research has found CBT can be effectively delivered by guided self-help and self-help methods. In contrast, there is less support for the effectiveness of pharmacotherapy alone as a treatment for BED. A major clinical challenge remains the need to help BED patients successfully lose weight and maintain the weight loss. Pressing research needs include developing treatments for those patients who fail to improve sufficiently with existing methods and finding ways to translate and disseminate effective treatments to practicing clinicians.

Obesity 6
Assessment and treatment

Introduction

Obesity is a serious and increasingly prevalent general medical condition that is now viewed as one of the major public health problems in the world. As summarized in chapter 2, obesity results from excess food intake relative to energy expenditure. Simply put, more calories are consumed than are burned off in daily life. Obesity is a markedly heterogeneous condition. As discussed earlier, the basic energy imbalance can occur from an array of complex genetic, biological, environmental, psychological, social, and behavioral factors that can differ across individuals and groups and even within individuals across the lifespan. With that context in mind, this chapter begins with an overview of the major assessment issues relevant to obesity. The major research findings about treatments and interventions will then be summarized.

The stigma of obesity

Rather than starting with the assessment of obesity by considering the core physical and medical aspects, this chapter will begin by first addressing the social and interpersonal context within which obese persons live. Obese persons face widespread stigma overtly and covertly. Biased attitudes toward overweight or obese persons begin at a very young age (Cramer & Steinwert, 1998; Goldfield & Chrisler, 1995; Hill & Silver, 1995; Kraig & Keel, 2001; Latner & Stunkard, 2003) and are evident throughout adulthood and across many different settings. Negative attitudes and weight bias toward the obese have been documented across education (Baum & Ford, 2004), employment (Baum & Ford, 2004), and social settings (Gortmaker, Must, Perrin, Sobol, & Dietz, 1993). Negative portrayals of the obese are frequent in the media (Geier, Schwartz, & Brownell, 2003; Greenberg, Eastin, Hofschire, Lachlan, & Brownell, 2003) and serve to perpetuate the negative "fat stereotypes." Recent research has demonstrated that such "anti-fat" biases are often internalized even among overweight persons (Wang, Brownell, & Wadden, 2004). Wang and colleagues (2004), using a performance-based test of bias to assess covert or implicit attitudes, observed that overweight persons have significant "anti-fat" views and stereotypes. The researchers noted that unlike other minority or discriminated groups, obese persons do not appear to hold positive views toward their obese peers.

The stigma associated with obesity may be getting worse. Latner and Stunkard (2003) recently replicated a famous study of stigma conducted in 1961 with children. In the original study, children were asked to rate or rank six different drawings of children with obesity, average weight, or various disabilities (including facial disfigurement, using crutches, using a wheelchair, and missing a hand). The same sets of instructions were given to 458 fifth and sixth graders by Latner and Stunkard (2003). The findings are summarized in Figure 6.1. As is evident from Figure 6.1, children in the original study and in the recent study conducted 40 years later ranked the drawing of the obese child the lowest. Furthermore, the ratings for the obese child were even lower now than 40 years ago, which is particularly striking when one considers that the rate of childhood obesity has more than doubled during the intervening time. These findings suggest that, despite the increase in prevalence of obesity, the stigma of obesity in children has increased over the past 40 years.

These negative biases have also been shown to exist among health professionals (Teachman & Brownell, 2001), including those who work specifically in the obesity field (Schwartz, Chambliss, Brownell, Blair, & Billington, 2003). Thus, it is possible that the stigma associated with obesity may negatively impact health-seeking behaviors and interactions with health care workers. Although obese women suffer from greater medical problems and utilize more health care than their leaner peers, obese women are less likely to seek preventive health care, and when they do they report frequently having negative experiences with health care professionals regarding the overweight (Drury & Louis, 2002; Fontaine, Faith, Allison, & Cheskin, 1998; Olson, Schumaker, & Yawn, 1994).

A recent survey found that while obese women were generally satisfied with medical care they received and with their physicians' medical expertise, they were much less satisfied with care received

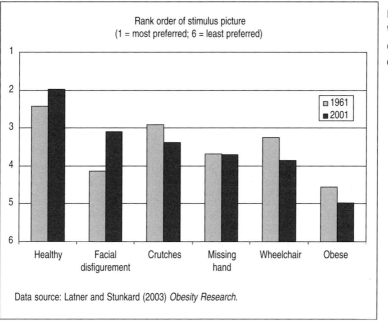

Rank order of stimulus picture
(1 = most preferred; 6 = least preferred)

□ 1961
■ 2001

Healthy   Facial   Crutches   Missing   Wheelchair   Obese
           disfigurement   hand

Data source: Latner and Stunkard (2003) *Obesity Research.*

Figure 6.1.
Worsening stigma of obesity among children.

for their overweight and with their physicians' knowledge of obesity (Wadden, Anderson, Foster, Bennett, Steinberg, & Sarwer, 2000). Another recent survey of 410 consecutive adult patients in two primary care practices revealed that most obese patients wanted substantially more help from their primary care doctors than they were receiving (Potter, Vu, & Croughan-Minihane, 2001). Whether these findings reflect negative views or discomfort in working with obese patients or insufficient expertise about weight control is uncertain. There are studies, however, that suggest that physicians' own weight status and views toward patients' weight status frequently result in less than optimal patient care (Anderson, Peterson, Fletcher, Mitchell, Thuras, & Crow, 2001; Perrin, Flower, & Ammerman, 2005). These findings challenge everyone to examine and become aware of their attitudes and behaviors towards obesity. The good news is that although negative associations exist, it appears that experiences in working with and caring for obese patients can contribute to reductions in the bias (Teachman & Brownell, 2001). It is important to bear in mind this social and interpersonal context (the stigma of obesity) throughout the processes of assessment and intervention.

Assessment and classification of obesity

The physical or medical assessment of obesity includes determination of body mass index (BMI), waist circumference, and overall medical risk. Obesity is defined as having a BMI (kg/m^2) of 30 or greater. Table 6.1 summarizes the classification of weight and obesity levels by the BMI. This classification, recommended by the NHLBI (1998a, 1998b) and WHO (1998), is currently viewed as the standard worldwide and has facilitated clinical and research communication. BMI is a better predictor of body fatness than body weight and correlates strongly (roughly 0.9) with expensive and cumbersome direct methods of measuring body composition (Lichtenbelt & Fogelholm, 1992). Some clinical judgment is indicated when using BMI. Most notably, BMI may overestimate obesity in athletes and muscular persons and may underestimate obesity in some older persons.

BMI classification and medical risk

The NHLBI (1998a, 1998b, 1998c) and WHO (1998) classification was based on morbidity and mortality findings from several longitudinal epidemiological studies. For example, analyses from the American Cancer Society Cohort Study, a prospective study of mortality in over one million people in the US started in 1982, revealed that a BMI between 23.5 and 24.9 had the lowest risk of death due to cardiovascular reasons (Calle, Thun, Petrelli, Rodriguez, & Heath, 1999). Analyses revealed that the risk for mortality from cardiovascular disease rose from BMI 25 to 29.9 and then rose very sharply for BMI greater than 30. Similar findings exist for other medical problems and causes of death. For example, the risk of type II diabetes begins to increase slightly at BMI of 24 in men and 22 in women, increases substantially at BMI greater than 25, and increases sharply at BMI above 30 (Chan, Rimm, Colditz, Stampfer, & Willett, 1994; Colditz, Willett, Rotnitzky, & Manson, 1995). An impressive body of data from the Harvard Alumni Study, the Health Professionals Follow-up Study, and the Nurse's Health Study converge in showing that overweight (defined as BMI $\geq$ 25) and especially obesity (BMI $\geq$ 30) are associated with increased risk for morbidity and mortality from multiple causes. The most recent analyses from the National Center for Health Statistics and the Centers for Disease Control (Flegal, Graubard, Williamson, & Gail, 2005) did not find that overweight was associated with excess mortality relative to normal weight but that

TABLE 6.1

Obesity classification by body mass index (BMI) and waist circumference (WC): Associated medical risk (relative to normal weight and waist)

Body mass index classification		Medical risk	
		Normal waist	High waist
Underweight	(< 18.5)		
Normal weight	(18.5–24.9)		Increased ??
Overweight	(25.0–29.9)	Increased	High
Obesity (Class I)	(30.0–34.9)	High	Very high
Obesity (Class II)	(35.0–39.9)	Very high	Very high
Extreme obesity (Class III)	(≥ 40.0)	Extremely high	Extremely high

Summary of medical risk by obesity level (BMI) and by abdominal obesity (waist circumference, WC). The medical risk (for type II diabetes, hypertension, and cardiovascular diseases) is relative to normal BMI and WC. High WC is defined as greater than 40 inches (102 centimeters) for men and greater than 35 inches (88 centimeters) for women. This summary is based on the (1998) report of the World Health Organization (WHO) and the National Health, Lung, and Blood Institute (NHLBI, 1998a, 1998b) guidelines.

obesity was strongly associated with excess mortality. Analyses have revealed that obesity shortens the lifespan (Fontaine et al., 2003).

Waist circumference classification and upper-body obesity

Excess abdominal fat (upper-body or android-type distribution) is associated with substantially greater morbidity and mortality than lower-body (gynoid-type) obesity. This observation dates back to Vague (1947) although it was not until definitive research published decades later that this became universally accepted. Excess abdominal fat is also an independent risk factor for morbidity and mortality, especially due to cardiovascular disease. Men are more likely than women to have abdominal fat distribution, but it is associated with increased medical problems regardless of gender. Waist circumference provides an adequate estimate of abdominal obesity, which would otherwise require expensive testing (Lichtenbelt & Fogelholm, 1992) and is a better predictor than the previously used waist-to-hip ratio. Despres (2002) and Depres, Moorjani, Lupien, Tremblay, Nadeau, & Bouchard, 1990) note, however, that waist and waist/hip measurements, while adequate for epidemiological studies, are more limited for clinical studies because they cannot distinguish between intra-abdominal fat (located in the abdominal cavity) and subcutaneous fat. Nonetheless, in addition to BMI, it is especially important to consider the distribution of abdominal fat as estimated by waist circumference. Table 6.1 summarizes obesity classification by BMI and waist circumference separately for men and women in terms of medical risk. The NHBLI (1998a, 1998b) notes some ethnic and age factors to consider when interpreting waist circumference and BMI. In persons of Asian descent, waist circumference is a better predictor than BMI of relative disease risk. In older persons, waist circumference is more important for estimating the risk of obesity-related medical problems.

Risk factors to consider

The NHLBI (1998a, 1998b) lists a number of risk factors to consider in overweight or obese persons. The risk factors and their defining levels are listed in Table 6.2. These risk factors for cardiovascular disease have been shown to substantially increase absolute risk. Of the risk factors listed, it should be noted that physical inactivity is associated with increased risk for both cardiovascular disease and for type II diabetes. Physical inactivity worsens the severity of the other risk factors listed and it is also an independent risk factor for mortality from cardiovascular diseases and from all causes. The NHLBI (1998a, 1998b) defined impaired fasting glucose (IFG) as between 110 and 125 mg/dL but it should be noted that the American Diabetes Association lowered the cutpoint for IFG (for "pre-diabetes") to 100 mg/dL. IFG is very well established as a risk factor for developing type II diabetes and appears to be an independent risk factor for cardiovascular disease.

Classification and treatment of obesity and overweight

The NHLBI (1998a, 1998b) guidelines recommend weight loss for persons classified as obese (BMI $\geq$ 30) and for persons classified as overweight (BMI $\geq$ 25–29.9) and who have two or more of the risk factors listed above. The federal guidelines also note that even modest weight loss (i.e., 5% to 10%) can substantially decrease the risk of developing obesity-related diseases. For persons who are overweight, do not have high waist circumference, and have fewer than two risk factors, prevention of further weight gain (rather than weight loss) is recommended.

TABLE 6.2

Risk factors to consider in overweight and obese persons

Risk factor	Defining level
High blood pressure (bp)	Systolic bp ≥ 140 mmHg; or diastolic bp ≥ 90 mmHg; or currently using anti-hypertensive medication
High low-density lipoprotein (LDL) cholesterol	≥ 160 mg/dL; or 130 to 159 mg/dL if two other risk factors
Low high-density lipoprotein (HDL) cholesterol	≥ 35 mg/dL
Impaired fasting glucose (IFG)	Fasting plasma glucose between 110 and 125 mg/dL (ADA (2004; ADA Expert Committee 2004) lowered level to ≥ 100)
Family history of premature coronary heart disease (CHD)	Heart attack or sudden death by first-degree male relative before 55 years of age or by first-degree female relative before 65 years of age
Age	≥ 45 for men or ≥ 55 (or postmenopausal) for women
Cigarette smoking	
Physical inactivity	

Medical assessment and co-morbidities

Since obesity is associated with a number of medical problems, assessment of those problems (most notably heart disease, athero-sclerotic disease, high blood pressure, diabetes, sleep apnea) is required and, if found, treatment is often indicated. As a general rule, increasing obesity, and especially waist circumference, is associated with greater risk for morbidity and mortality. The most serious and common problems associated with obesity are listed in Table 6.3, although this does not represent an exhaustive listing of the many bodily systems and health problems negatively impacted by obesity. Major issues about these medical problems are briefly noted below.

Coronary heart disease

As noted elsewhere in this text, obesity is associated with elevated rates of morbidity and mortality due to coronary heart disease as well as due to "all causes." It was not until the late 1990s that obesity became considered an "independent" risk factor for heart disease by

TABLE 6.3

Common medical problems associated with obesity

- Coronary heart (cardiovascular) disease
- Type II (non-insulin-dependent) diabetes mellitus
- Stroke
- Hypertension
- Dyslipidemia
- Cancer
- Respiratory
- Gallbladder
- Arthritis

the American Heart Association (Eckel & Krauss, 1998). Since obesity is so strongly associated with other medical problems, such as diabetes, hypertension, and dyslipidemia, which are each strong independent risk factors for heart disease, there existed some controversy about how important the specific effects of obesity were for heart disease. Longer term findings from the major longitudinal studies and further consideration of the complexities of combining different risk factors when predicting health outcomes suggest obesity is a major and independent risk factor for heart disease (Eckel & Krauss, 1998) and excess mortality (Flegal et al., 2005).

Diabetes

Type II (non-insulin-dependent) diabetes is strongly associated with obesity. The risk of type II diabetes begins to increase slightly at BMI of 24 in men and 22 in women, increases substantially at BMI greater than 25, and increases very sharply at BMI above 30 (Chan et al., 1994; Colditz et al., 1995). Greater obesity and longer duration of being obese are associated with diabetes.

Roughly 8.7% (18 million people) of adults (aged 20 or older) in the United States have diabetes (ADA, 2004; ADA Expert Committee, 2004) which is strongly associated with heightened morbidity and mortality, particularly by heart disease (Hu, Stampfer, Haffner, Solomon, Willett, & Manson, 2002). The economic and health costs associated with diabetes are staggering and have been estimated to be over $132 billion in total costs (ADA, 2004; ADA Expert Committee, 2004). Obesity, which has comparable direct costs to type II diabetes, also accounts for roughly 60% of the direct costs due to diabetes (Wolf & Colditz, 1998).

Research using data from the Nurses Health Study has revealed that an elevated risk of coronary heart disease is evident *before* or prior to a clinical diagnosis of type II diabetes (Hu et al., 2002). These and other findings have led to recent emphasis on identifying pre-diabetes (persons at increased risk for developing diabetes) at an even earlier stage. Pre-diabetes is determined based on either having impaired fasting glucose (IFG; newly revised criteria of 100–125 mg/dL) or impaired gluocose tolerance (IGT; criteria remain unchanged and are 140–199 mg/dL) (ADA, 2004; ADA Expert Committee, 2004). Recently released estimates, based on this revised definition for pre-diabetes (IFG 100–125 mg/dL), are that 40% of US adults aged 40 to 74 (41 million people) have this condition which greatly increases their risk of developing type II diabetes within ten years (ADA, 2004; ADA Expert Committee, 2004).

Both pre-diabetes and diabetes are increasing in prevalence, in large part due to the increases in obesity. The public health impact of intervening at the pre-diabetic level has been demonstrated convincingly in two landmark studies, the United States Diabetes Prevention Program (DPP; DPRG, 2002) and the Finnish Diabetes Prevention Program (Tuomilehto et al., 2001). The DPP (DPRG, 2002), for example, demonstrated that the progression to type II diabetes is not inevitable and that modest weight loss with lifestyle interventions and physical activity reduced the development of type II diabetes by 58% over three years. Thus, the interventions for obesity described later in this chapter, even if they produce only modest weight loss, can potentially have profound personal and public health impact on both obesity and major associated co-morbidities.

Hypertension

In general, the higher the weight and the longer the duration of being overweight, the greater the chance of developing hypertension (generally considered to be a problem if blood pressure is greater than 140/90 mmHg). Rates of hypertension in overweight persons tend to be at least twice that of non-overweight persons (Higgins, Kannel, Garrison, Pinsky, & Stokes, 1988). For every 20 pound increase in body weight, the average increase in blood pressure (systolic/diastolic) is 3/2 mm/Hg. As for other problems, abdominal fatness is a more important contributor than lower body fatness to hypertension.

Dyslipidemia

Dyslipidemia refers to abnormalities in lipids circulating throughout the blood stream. Three concerns tend to be: (1) high triglyceride levels; (2) low levels of high-density lipoprotein cholesterol (HDL); (3) high levels of low-density lipoprotein (LDL). These abnormal levels increase atherosclerotic disease and risk for coronary heart disease.

Other medical issues

There are many other health problems and serious diseases that co-occur in obesity. Obesity is clearly associated with increased risk for some cancers (e.g., endometrial, cervical, ovarian, gallbladder). Various respiratory problems are common in obese persons. One of the most common respiratory problems that develops with obesity is sleep apnea. Less common but severe respiratory problems can result in pulmonary hypertension and heart failure. As expected, arthritis and degenerative joint disease are common in older and heavier persons. Gallbladder disease and gallstones are common in obese persons, particularly women. Here it is important to note that gall-stones are a common problem in cases with rapid and large weight losses.

The metabolic syndrome

The metabolic syndrome refers to a clustering of cardiovascular disease risk factors associated with abdominal obesity. Overall, the metabolic syndrome is increasing in prevalence and the prevalence increases considerably with age: 45% of persons aged 60 to 69 versus 20% in persons aged 40 to 49 (Ford, Giles, & Dietz, 2002). This concept has evolved from a syndrome described by Kylin in 1923 (initially comprising hypertension, hyperglycemia, and gout) and by Reaven in 1988 as "Syndrome X" and was renamed the "metabolic syn-drome" by the WHO in 1998 (as detailed in Isomaa et al., 2001). In 2001, the National Cholesterol Education Program (NCEP), Adult Treatment Panel (ATP) III published their definition of the metabolic syndrome and guidelines. Table 6.4 provides a summary of risk factors for the metabolic syndrome and their defining levels provided separately for men and women. At least three of the five criteria must be met for the diagnosis of the metabolic syndrome. The defining levels noted in Table 6.4 contain one noteworthy revision. Instead of the impaired fasting glucose level of 110 mg/dL adopted by the NCEP, a level of 100 mg/dL is listed to reflect the American Diabetes

TABLE 6.4

The metabolic syndrome

Risk factor	Defining level	
	Men	Women
Abdominal obesity (waist circumference)	> 102 cm (> 40 in)	> 88 cm (> 35 in)
Triglycerides	≥ 150 mg/dL	≥ 150 mg/dL
HDL-cholesterol	< 40 mg/dL	< 50 mg/dL
Blood pressure	≥ 130/85 mmHg	≥ 130/85 mmHg
Fasting glucose	≥ 100 mg/dL	≥ 100 mg/dL

Summary of risk factors for the metabolic syndrome and their defining levels provided separately for men and women. At least three of the five criteria must be met for the diagnosis of the metabolic syndrome.

These guidelines are based on the National Cholesterol Education Program (NCEP, 2001) Expert Panel on Detection, Evaluation, and Treatment of High Blood Cholesterol in Adults (Adult Treatment Panel III; ATP III) report published in the *Journal of the American Medical Association*. The summary provided above contains one noteworthy revision. Given the recommendation by the American Diabetes Association in 2003 to lower the criterion of impaired fasting glucose from 110 mg/dL and the notation of this change by a panel of experts at a meeting convened to address this definition (Grundy, Brewer, Cleeman, Smith, & Lenfant, 2004) the lower criterion is noted.

Association lowering the criterion from 110 mg/dL in 2003 and the subsequent notation of this change by a panel of experts at another NECP meeting (Grundy et al., 2004).

Assessment of non-medical factors associated with obesity

An overview of assessment of non-medical factors associated with obesity follows. As noted above, it is important to be sensitive to the strong social stigma faced by obese persons in many settings. It is also important to be sensitive to patients' frustrations regarding previous unsuccessful "diets" (Brownell & Rodin, 1994). Another challenge is the nearly universal existence of unrealistic weight loss goals and expectations held by obese persons seeking treatment (Foster, Wadden, Vogt, & Brewer, 1997b; Masheb & Grilo, 2002; Wadden, Womble, Sarwer, Berkowitz, Clark, & Foster, 2003).

Studies have found that obese patients who seek treatment frequently have weight loss expectations that greatly exceed the potential results of any current obesity treatments (except for surgery). In these studies, patients' reports of their ideal weight loss translate to an average of about 35% reduction in their current weight. One study found that such "ideal" weight loss goals expressed by obese patients tend to be very close to their lowest adult weight ever (Masheb & Grilo, 2002). Perhaps more importantly, patients' reports of what their "disappointed" weight would be following treatment translate to an average of roughly 15% reduction in their current weight. This 15% reduction (which is viewed as disappointing by obese patients) is roughly twice as much as most obesity treatments can produce (summarized below). Such weight loss expectations are greater than the current expert recommendations of establishing realistic goals for weight losses as little as 5% to 10%. Such modest weight losses may result in significant health improvements (Blackburn 1995; Goldstein, 1992) and psychosocial well-being (Wadden, Steen, Wingate, & Foster, 1996). Interestingly, the health improvements from such modest weight losses are often most evident in obese patients with more risk factors. Nonetheless, such weight losses are certainly cosmetically and psychologically disappointing to the majority of obese patients entering treatment. Obesity experts have increasingly urged professionals working with obese patients to encourage setting modest and realistic goals. Greater attention needs to be paid to the multiple benefits (e.g., health, fitness, psychological benefits) of changes – instead of the traditional focus on weight loss per se. Getting obese patients to shift expectations has been difficult (Wadden et al., 2003).

Psychological functioning

Despite the stigma and negative views towards obese persons, a very large body of research has found that obese and non-obese persons differ little in psychological and psychiatric functioning (Friedman & Brownell, 1995). If the two extremes of weight are excluded (i.e., anorexia nervosa and extreme obesity), obese and non-obese people generally show very similar rates of psychological and psychiatric disorders. Research has found two important exceptions. Most studies have found that obese persons suffer from greater body image dissatisfaction and some studies have found that obese persons may have lower self-esteem (Friedman & Brownell, 1995). A more important issue than trying to identify between-group differences (obese versus non-obese) is to understand within-group differences and variability in needs.

Body image concerns are common in obese persons. Interestingly, less attention has been devoted to body image in treatment research with obese persons than in the area of eating disorders. Body image and appearance concerns are major reasons (along with health issues) for seeking treatment by obese persons and by obese persons with BED (Reas, Masheb, & Grilo, 2004). Although body image concerns in the obese are frequently distressing and often of longstanding nature, such concerns (unlike the overevaluation of weight and shape that characterize eating disorders) seem to improve substantially with weight loss.

Body image in obese patients has been found to improve substantially across a variety of obesity treatments regardless of whether the interventions included a cognitive aspect or a body image component. For example, Foster, Wadden, and Vogt (1997a) reported that body image improved substantially in obese women during behavioral weight loss treatment and the improvements in body image were both unrelated to the amount of weight loss and were sustained after treatment despite some weight regain. Wadden and colleagues (2004) reported substantial improvements in body image among obese women who received three very different dieting interventions. Sorbara and Geliebter (2002) reported substantial improvements in body image in obese men and women participating in a low-calorie liquid formula diet, although those patients with an early onset of obesity seemed to improve less than those patients who became obese as adults.

Of particular relevance here is the recent resurgence in research attention being paid to disordered eating in obese persons (Tanofsky-Kraff & Yanovski, 2004). As reviewed in chapter 5, obese persons who binge eat represent a subgroup of obese patients characterized by higher rates of associated problems across diverse areas than obese persons who do not binge eat (Grilo, 1998). Binge eating in the obese is associated with substantially elevated levels of psychiatric problems as well as with elevated psychological distress (Grilo, 1998; Yanovski et al., 1993). In addition, among obese persons who binge eat there is a subgroup characterized by strong negative affect (Grilo et al., 2001a; Stice, Agras, Telch, Halmi, Mitchell, & Wilson, 2001). This subtype (labeled dietary-negative affect type) has higher levels of associated eating and psychological disturbance than the more "pure" dietary subtype. Obese patients with binge eating problems are believed to require treatments that address these broad problem areas (Goldfein et al., 2000). Those treatment models and findings were reviewed in chapter 5. It is worth noting here that the issue of whether obese persons who binge eat require different treatments from non-binge eaters is not without controversy (Devlin et al., 2005; Gladis et al., 1998b; Sherwood et al., 1999).

Eating behaviors and nutrition

Research has demonstrated how poorly individuals report their eating behaviors. These limitations seem to be present across different methods of reporting. Although self-monitoring and use of daily food records reduces some of the biases and limitations in retrospective recall (Grilo et al., 2001b, 2001c; Wilson & Vitousek, 1999), research has found that even these methods can result in underestimates. In general, most individuals underestimate how much they eat (Asbeck, Mast, Bierwag, Westenhofer, Acheson, & Muller, 2002; McKenzie, Johnson, Harvey-Berino, & Gold, 2002; Scagliusi, Polacow, Artioli, Benatti, & Lancha, 2003). Although both thin and overweight persons tend to underestimate caloric intake, the degree of underestimation is generally greater among obese persons (Lichtman et al., 1992). Lichtman and colleagues (1992), for example, found that obese persons who were reported to be "diet resistant" (i.e., persons for whom dieting was ineffective and presumably due to slow metabolism) actually had resting metabolic rates and total energy expenditures within 5% of predicted values for their body composition. In contrast to the apparent lack of an abnormal metabolism, these obese persons were found to underestimate by 47% the amount of food they ate and overestimate by 51% the amount of physical activity they performed during a two-week period. These findings, obtained with sophisticated measurements of energy expenditure (doubly labeled water technique), have been generally confirmed in other studies (Buhl, Gallagher, Hoy, Matthews, & Heymsfield, 1995). Thus, the failure to lose weight or to sustain weight loss may be due to the basic formula of overeating and underactivity.

Although some of the error in estimating eating and exercise is likely due to social desirability or embarrassment, other factors cannot be discounted. Clinically, it seems that the inconvenience of detailed record keeping and straightforward error or lack of knowledge about portion sizes are also contributors to such inaccurate reporting. The implication is that clinicians and researchers working in these areas need to sensitively address these issues. It seems important to devote time to provide detailed descriptions of portion sizes and calories in different foods along with the value of careful record keeping (Scagliusi et al., 2003; Wilson & Vitousek, 1999). This basic challenge is evident even from self-report and survey data. For example, Bish and colleagues (2005), using data from the Behavioral Risk Factor Surveillance System, a telephone-based survey of 184,450 adults conducted in 2000, observed that although 46% of women and 33% of men reported that they were trying to lose weight, only 19% of women and 22% of men reported that they were eating fewer calories and using at least 150 minutes weekly of leisure-time physical activity.

Overview of treatment for obesity

There exists a very broad range of interventions and treatments for obesity. Over the years, treatments of varied types and intensity have been developed. While many have been attempted, few have received careful research attention. Treatments have ranged from pure self-help and low intensity commercial self-help programs to high intensity and invasive medical procedures including various forms of surgery. This review will focus primarily on those treatment approaches that have received the most study (behavioral treatments, very-low-calorie diets, pharmacotherapy, and surgery). In addition, a brief overview of what is currently known about self-help and commercial weight loss programs will be provided since millions of Americans enroll in such programs every year (Tsai & Wadden, 2005).

Before discussing the different treatments, it is important to note several points about context. Selecting a treatment for oneself or prescribing a treatment for a patient is complex. Obesity is heterogeneous and the needs of individuals vary greatly (Brownell & Wadden, 1991). It is unlikely that any one treatment approach will meet everyone's needs. Risk-benefit ratios should be considered when thinking about treatment options. Here it is critical to bear in mind that not pursuing treatment for obesity has risk. So, the risks associated with some of the treatments that will be described must be weighed against both the potential benefit of improvement while keeping in mind the risk associated with doing nothing. The severity of the condition is also an important factor. For example, a moderately obese patient with significant obesity-related health problems would warrant consideration of more aggressive and comprehensive treatment (including possibly medication and surgery) than would a slightly overweight person with no co-existing medical conditions or other risk factors.

Overall, research on the treatment of obesity (except for surgery) can be summarized as follows. Many but not all approaches can produce significant short-term weight loss. For many patients, however, the weight loss is difficult to maintain over time and most of it is usually regained within a few years. For many, the amount of weight loss – although modest and cosmetically short of patients' goals – if it could somehow be maintained, could have potential medical benefits, especially for the patients with greater health risks. A more detailed review of the major approaches follows.

Self-help and commercial weight loss programs

From an intensity or step-care perspective, pure self-help and commercial weight loss programs represent the first and second steps, respectively, of a general four-step model for obesity treatment (NHLBI, 1998a, 1998b). It seems that diet, nutritional, and exercise products are everywhere one looks and that comments about "dieting" are ubiquitous. It is difficult, however, to really know how many people are currently trying to follow a pure self-help program for weight control. The most recent data from the Behavioral Risk Factor Surveillance System in 2000 suggested that 46% of women and 33% of men were trying to lose weight (Bish et al., 2005), but how many are actually following some program is uncertain. There are anecdotal reports for obesity, like other problems such as smoking, that many persons are quite successful on their own. With that context, what do we know about self-help and commercial weight loss programs other than that they enroll millions and tend to be profitable year after year?

Tsai and Wadden (2005) recently completed a systematic and careful review of the major commercial weight loss programs in the US. Studies were identified that included two non-profit self-help programs (Overeaters Anonymous, Take Off Pounds Sensibly), and the following commercial weight loss programs: non-medical diet programs (e.g., Weight Watchers, Jenny Craig, LA Weight Loss), very-low-calorie diets (non-university based), medically based diet programs (Optifast, Health Management Resources), and internet-based programs (eDiets). Minimal study criteria were used including the requirement of at least 10 patients, 12 weeks of duration, and the study used the same basic program given to the public.

The major finding of the Tsai and Wadden (2005) review was the dearth of good quality studies on these approaches. Most of the studies had high dropout rates and reported data that are probably best interpreted as the best-case scenario because analyses rarely included the dropouts. The organized self-help programs and the commercial internet programs resulted in minimal weight loss. Only three studies existed for the very-low-calorie diets and medically based commercial programs, and only one was a controlled study (Anderson, Brinkman-Kaplan, Hamilton, Logan, Collins, & Gustafson, 1994). These programs, which involved considerable fees, reported roughly 15% to 25% weight losses for patients who complete treatments. However, these programs had very high dropout rates and most patients regained 50% or more of the weight within two years.

Of the widely used commercial diet programs, Tsai and Wadden (2005) were able to locate studies only for Weight Watchers. At the time, Weight Watchers had been tested in three randomized controlled trials, one of which was a large study of obese men and women with two-year follow-up (Heshka et al., 2003). In the study by Heshka and colleagues (2003), nearly 75% of participants completed the two-year study. A conservative comparison considering all patients who began treatments revealed that patients following the Weight Watchers program lost more weight than those following self-help after one year (4.3 kg versus 1.3 kg) and two years (2.9 kg versus 0.2 kg). Waist circumference and BMI also decreased more in this commercial diet than in the self-help condition. This study suggests that this one commercial program is superior to a self-help approach, but the weight loss achieved is minimal. It seems important that obese patients who consider or seek such commercial weight loss programs become aware that they have not been carefully studied and the few available studies are not particularly encouraging.

More recently, a randomized controlled study has been published that directly compared four popular diets (Weight Watchers, Atkins, Zone, Ornish). It is important to note that the study was compared at an academic medical center and thus it may not represent how the programs are typically delivered to the public by non-professionals. Overall dietary adherence was low and dropout rates were fairly high and as follows: 50% for Ornish, 47% for Atkins, 35% for Zone, and 35% for Weight Watchers. Average weight losses after one year, which were modest, did not differ significantly for the different diet programs and were as follows: 3.3 kg for Ornish, 2.1 kg for Atkins, 3.2 kg for Zone, and 3.0 kg for Weight Watchers. The weight losses for those patients who did not drop out and completed the programs were slightly better. An important finding was that while weight loss was not associated with diet type, it was significantly associated with self-reported dietary adherence. So, patients who reported they were trying to adhere to their diet goals lost more weight.

Very-low-calorie diets

Very-low-calorie diets (VLCD) were widely used and tested during the 1980s and early 1990s (Wadden, Van Itallie, & Blackburn, 1990). VLCDs involve fasting (calorie levels generally between 400 and 800 kcal/day) with protein supplements. In general, VLCDs produce rapid and significant weight losses but research has found that these weight losses tend to be poorly maintained. Studies found that combining behavior therapy with VLCDs decreases weight regain during the year following the use of the VLCD but several studies that followed patients for three to five years found that all of the weight lost was eventually regained (Wadden, Stunkard, & Liebschutz, 1988; Wadden, Sternberg, Letizia, Stunkard, & Foster, 1989). Wadden, Foster, and Letizia (1994) found that the combination of a VLCD and behavior therapy had no long-term advantage over the combination of a conventional balanced moderate deficit diet plus behavior therapy. Variations of these VLCDs are currently in use and available via a variety of commercial programs (Optifast, Health Management Resources) which, as reviewed above, have little to no support (Tsai & Wadden, 2005).

Behavioral treatment

Early forms of behavior therapy focused primarily on changing specific eating behaviors and were conducted alongside nutritional and exercise interventions. These practices evolved over the years (Wilson, 1994) and today behavioral therapies have generally integrated important dietary and exercise components into a more holistic approach (e.g., Brownell, 2000). These behavioral treatments typically include modest dietary restriction (goals of 1200–1500 kcal/day) with an emphasis on behavioral strategies to help limit intake and increase activity.

Behavioral treatments for obesity, particularly from professionally directed programs in specialty clinics or university settings, have been studied extensively. Numerous critical reviews have reported fairly consistent overall conclusions (Brownell & Jeffery, 1987; Wilson, 1994). Most behavioral treatments produce significant short-term weight losses, but are characterized by gradual and continuous weight regain after treatment. During the first year after treatment, patients tend to regain, on average, one-third to one-half of the weight they lost, and most patients regain their entire weight loss by five years (Kramer, Jeffery, Forster, & Snell, 1989).

Prevention of relapse (Brownell & Wadden, 1992) and improving maintenance (Perri, McAllister, Gange, Jordon, McAdoo, Nezu, 1988; Perri, Nezu, & Viegener, 1992) have been viewed as the primary challenge in obesity treatment for the past two decades. Treatments have become longer as they have tried to de-emphasize simplistic acute care or short-term approaches while emphasizing the need for ongoing or lifestyle change. Such lifestyle views and relapse prevention techniques have become standard components in established treatment manuals (e.g., Brownell, 2000). Treatments now produce slightly more weight loss, but the increases in weight losses are primarily a function of the longer treatment rather than of more potent treatments (Brownell & Jeffery, 1987; Wilson, 1994). Nonetheless, it cannot be emphasized enough that since obesity is now regarded as a chronic problem, it makes sense to view ongoing long-term approaches as a required philosophy (i.e., there are no "quick fixes").

Nutritional and dietary components

There is considerable variation across weight control programs in the nature of their nutritional and caloric recommendations. Most established behavioral programs recommend roughly 1200 to 1500 kcal/day goals. Such modest caloric goals result in enough energy deficit to result in gradual and safe weight loss for most people. There are several challenges, however, in achieving this seemingly straightforward goal. When many people start weight control programs, they are very eager to see rapid and large results and may become impatient with this approach. A different and more complicated challenge is that 1200 to 1500 kcal is actually much less food than most people realize. Even with careful and ongoing attention to food records, clinical and research experience suggests that obese persons under-report and substantially underestimate food intake. There is reason to believe that this underestimation of food intake is a much greater problem now than it was 20 years ago. As discussed in chapter 2, typical serving sizes across nearly every type of food have grown steadily. So a typical bagel today, which is twice or three times larger than 20 years ago, may actually represent three (not one) servings.

Given gender, ethnicity, age, and individual differences in metabolic processes and energy expenditure, Grilo and Brownell (1998, 2001) recommended the following general approach to estimate calorie goals for a patient to achieve a modest deficit. Begin with a 1500 kcal/day goal for men and a 1200 kcal/day goal for women and carefully record all food intake in a food diary. Given the continuously increasing serving sizes in our society, it is important to find ways to record actual sizes of the foods consumed. By keeping track of weight changes over time, these careful food records can be used to help make adjustments in types and quantities of food necessary to accomplish ongoing weight loss goals. This approach assumes that there will be variability between individuals and within individuals over time due to changes in water loss, metabolic shifts, lean tissue loss, and changes in activity levels. This approach can lead to a more collaborative process between the professional and the patient and will produce a more individualized and accurate caloric estimate.

Nutrition amount and balance: The Food Guide Pyramid

In addition to total caloric intake, obesity treatments must consider balanced nutrition practices. The Food Guide Pyramid published by the US Department of Agriculture is now widely disseminated on many food packages. The Food Guide Pyramid shows recommended dietary guidelines with clearly specified daily servings for all five food groups. Roughly, these federal guidelines suggest limiting dietary fat to less than 30% of total daily intake, with roughly 50% of total intake coming from carbohydrates and 20% from protein.

The developers of the Food Guide Pyramid had hoped for this basic information to be easily understood. It has become evident, however, that the concept of "servings" has greatly limited the usefulness of this method for promoting dietary guidelines. The portion sizes of nearly all foods and beverages have grown dramatically during the past two decades (Astrup, 2005). The portion sizes that people have become accustomed to are much larger (and with far greater calories) than the federal guidelines regarding serving sizes. In April 2005, a revised Food Guide Pyramid was published by the US Department of Agriculture and Centers for Disease Control. The revised version of the Food Guide Pyramid has two important revisions. First, it attempts to provide nutritional recommendations by relying on more "typical" portion and food servings in current use. Second, it now includes a physical activity component, to convey the importance of overall energy balance. In the revised Food Guide Pyramid, persons who are less active are provided with more modest food intake goals.

Alternative nutritional approaches

Optimal dietary and nutritional composition has become a source of considerable debate. In large part this has been triggered by the widespread use of various self-help and commercial diet plans advocating seemingly imbalanced and extreme diets (e.g., high protein/low carbohydrate diets). In response to concerns about such diets and their widespread commercial use, a number of recent studies have compared low fat diets to low carbohydrate/high protein diets or portion-control popular diets (Foster et al. 2003; Samaha et al., 2003; Stern et al., 2004; Yancy, Olsen, Guyton, Bakst, & Westman, 2004). These studies reported fairly high dropout rates (generally over one-third of patients) and concerns regarding dietary adherence. In these studies, in comparison to conventional low fat diets, the low carbohydrate diets were found to produce similar weight loss in one study (Stern et al., 2004), significantly greater weight loss in another study (Yancy et al., 2004), and greater weight loss at 6 months but not at 12 months (Foster et al., 2003). Surprisingly, these studies found significantly greater improvements in some of the obesity-related risk factors for the low carbohydrate than the low fat diets. These studies provide some support for the short-term safety and potential effectiveness of low carbohydrate diets and highlight the need for continued and longer term research. Stern and colleagues (2004) concluded that these findings suggest that limiting carbohydrates in obese persons, who might be overeating carbohydrates, may result in some positive metabolic improvements along with the modest weight loss. A different approach to both the nutritional issues and to the challenge of portion control is the use of "meal replacements." A variety of low calorie meal replacements are widely sold but it remains uncertain how helpful they are. A recent critical review of the emerging literature, which pooled findings from six controlled trials, concluded that these types of interventions can safely and effectively produce weight loss (Heymsfield, van Mierlo, van der Knaap, & Frier, 2003). More recent studies have reported further support for the potential utility of meal replacements within the context of behavioral weight loss interventions (Hannum et al., 2004; Poston et al., 2005).

Adherence and dietary intake: What do controlled experiments tell us?

The preceding overview of nutritional and dietary intake issues highlights the key elements of adherence and compliance. Many of the studies reviewed above indicate concerns about the level of adherence to dietary prescriptions. This represents a major limitation in the body of research and needs to be kept in mind when interpreting the studies. As noted above, many people are inaccurate reporters of calories and of food intake. This raises the logical question of whether the failure to lose weight or improve metabolic profile is due to biological resistances to weight loss ("dieting resistance," "low metabolism"), to specific characteristics or limitations of the weight loss program, or to poor compliance. Two controlled experiments will be described that address different aspects of these issues.

Behavioral reasons for poor outcomes

Smith and Wing (1991) compared weight losses achieved during two consecutive VLCDs. This study was performed to test various possible explanations for a common observation that dieters frequently achieved less weight loss during a second trial of a VLCD than the first time on a similar diet. Since the VLCDs involve very low caloric intakes using specific food products, it was assumed that some type of metabolic shift must have occurred with the repeated dieting that made it harder to lose weight. Forty-five obese patients with type II diabetes were enrolled in a 52-week behavioral program that incorporated a strict VLCD (400 to 500 kcal/day) for two 12-week periods (weeks 1 to 12 and weeks 28 to 40).

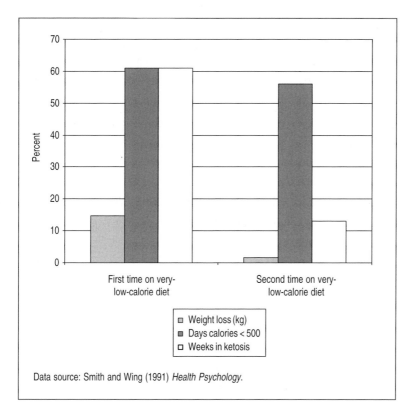

Data source: Smith and Wing (1991) *Health Psychology.*

Figure 6.2.
First and second time on very-low-calorie diets: Weight change and adherence measures.

Figure 6.2 summarizes the findings from the Smith and Wing (1991) study. Weight losses achieved during the first VLCD were substantially greater than during the second VLCD (average weight losses of 15.5 kg versus 1.4 kg, respectively). Careful assessments, however, revealed that this failure to achieve weight loss during the second VLCD was due to poor adherence. As shown in Figure 6.2, patients' self-reports of following the 500 kcal/day VLCD did not drop off much from the first to the second VLCD. Patients self-reported being compliant on 62% and 57% of the days, respectively. In sharp contrast, lab tests revealed that patients were in ketosis (a metabolic state reflecting caloric restriction) for 61% of the days during the first VLCD versus only 13% during the second VLCD. This study cannot address the reasons for the inaccurate reporting of food intake during the second VLCD. It is, however, a convincing demonstration that behavioral factors and compliance explain poor results on a repeated diet and that patients' self-reports of adherence can be greatly biased.

High fat versus low fat

In chapter 2, the association between eating high fat foods and increasing obesity and body fat was discussed. The findings from initial treatment studies comparing low carbohydrate to high carbohydrate diets reviewed above (Foster et al. 2003; Samaha et al., 2003; Stern et al., 2004; Yancy et al., 2004) appear to be at odds with common sense and with the well-established findings noted previously in chapter 2. It is possible that eating too many calories comprised of high fat foods may produce obesity, but that limiting calories per se (regardless of whether by low carbohydrate or high carbohydrate diets) can produce weight loss. The poor adherence noted in the treatment studies and the significant limitations in self-report of food intake, particularly when having limited success, dictate the need for carefully conducted experimental work to address such questions.

Laboratory studies with animal models offer powerful solutions to such clinical problems. Petro and colleagues (2004) fed B6 mice (a specific strain of mice highly susceptible to diabetes and obesity) three specific diets for 11 weeks in a highly controlled laboratory environment. This experiment used four-week-old male B6 mice who were kept individually in a carefully controlled environment for temperature and light/dark cycles. The three diets were exactly prepared and included: low fat diet fed ad libitum (LF; i.e., free feeding with access to food); high fat diet fed ad libitum (HF); or a high fat restricted caloric diet (HF-R). The HF-R mice ate an average of 726 kcal per day, which did not differ from the LF mice which ate an average of 719 kcal (despite no restriction); both of these levels were significantly lower than the average of 879 kcal consumed by the HF. Thus, the HF mice ate substantially more calories than the HF-R and both those groups ate more fat (but not calories) than the LF mice. The major findings for body weight and body fat are summarized in Figure 6.3. As is evident from Figure 6.3, high fat intake has an independent (added) effect on increasing both body weight and body fatness. Importantly, glucose levels were significantly increased in mice fed both the high fat diets. Petro and colleagues (2004) concluded that reducing the total number of calories from a high fat diet lowers but does not prevent the development of excess fatness or diabetes in the B6 mouse.

Of course, many different animal models exist that vary in susceptibility to obesity. This particular model was selected specifically because it is susceptible to developing obesity and

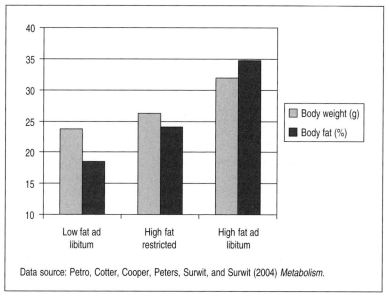

Figure 6.3.
The effects of three
diets on mice:
Importance of both
calories and fat.

Data source: Petro, Cotter, Cooper, Peters, Surwit, and Surwit (2004) *Metabolism*.

diabetes in response to diet. This model seems most relevant to human obesity and the metabolic syndrome. Caution is indicated when attempting to generalize findings from animal models to humans. In this case, however, and in contrast to the recent marginal findings for the various fad diets, there are clear findings from earlier treatment studies suggesting that obese patients are more successful in maintaining weight loss on low fat/high carbohydrate ad libitum than on more conventional but calorie restricted diets (Toubro & Astrup, 1997). These findings suggest that lower fat diets result in lower body weight and body fat.

Exercise and physical activity

Exercise predicts successful weight loss maintenance

Physical activity is an essential component of any obesity treatment program (Grilo, 1994; Grilo et al., 1993). Physical activity alone without significant dietary change is usually not enough to produce significant weight loss in most obese persons. The combination of exercise and diet, although not consistently associated with weight loss in the short term, is frequently associated with successful weight loss maintenance across diverse groups of obese adults (Andersen,

Wadden, Bartlett, Zemel, Verde, & Franckowiak, 1999; Bryner, Toffle, Ulrich, & Yeater, 1997) and children (Epstein, Wing, Koeske, & Valoski, 1984) and with very different forms of diets (Pavlou, Krey, & Steffee, 1989).

Exercise predicts health

In addition to predicting weight loss, increased physical activity and fitness are consistently associated with improved health and decreased mortality (Barlow, Kohl, Gibbons, & Blair, 1995; Lee, Jackson, & Blair, 1998; Pate et al., 1995). Physical activity may be particularly beneficial for obese persons with elevated risk factors or with obesity-related medical problems (Helmrich, Ragland, Leung, & Paffenbarger, 1991; Kanaley, Andersen-Reid, Oenning, Kottke, & Jensen, 1993). There is evidence suggesting that exercise can improve health even when little weight loss occurs (Wing, Koeske, Epstein, Nowalk, Gooding, & Becker, 1987; Wood, Stefanick, Williams, & Haskell, 1991). Although there continues to be controversy regarding how much and what type of exercise is best for weight loss, there is evidence that even modest levels of physical activity can be sufficient to improve health in many persons (Barlow et al., 1995; Duncan, Gordon, & Scott, 1991; Rippe, Ward, Porcari, & Freedson, 1988). Lastly, fitness protects against health risks even in overweight persons (Barlow et al., 1995; Lee et al., 1998).

What kind and how much exercise?

Considerable research has attempted to provide guidance around issues of optimal exercise prescription (intensity levels, frequency, types of approaches, etc.). For example, research has considered intermittent versus traditional continuous exercise (Jakicic, Winters, Lang, & Wing, 1999), different forms of exercise such as aerobic and strength training in different combinations (Wadden et al., 1997), advantages of home versus in-group (Perri, Martin, Leermakers, Sears, & Notelovitz, 1997), and lifestyle versus structured exercise (Andersen et al., 1999; Dunn, Marcus, Kampert, Garcia, Kohl, & Blair, 1999). Strong debate continues. Some experts recommend modest cumulative lifestyle physical activity while others stress the need for improving fitness. Wing (1999) and others have urged reconsideration of exercise prescriptions in light of findings suggesting that higher levels (i.e., 2500 kcal/week) are stronger predictors of successful weight maintenance. Nonetheless, given the general consensus that consistency is the key to long-term success, many experts still advocate that obese persons aim to accumulate at least 30 minutes of some form of physical activity on at least five days of every week.

Lifestyle physical activity

Controlled treatment studies have found that interventions fostering lifestyle physical activity may be as effective as traditional structured exercise programs. Andersen and colleagues (1999) reported that adding lifestyle exercise versus structured exercise to a comprehensive behavior therapy program resulted in comparable positive improvements in obese women. Dunn and colleagues (1999) found that lifestyle exercise and a structured exercise program resulted in similar overall increases in physical activity, and improved cardio-respiratory fitness and blood pressure in previously sedentary but healthy adults. Thus, lifestyle physical activity, which is associated with fewer injuries and less cost, may be an effective way for preventing weight gain, losing weight, and improving health.

Pharmacotherapy

What role for medication?

It is not acceptable to try to treat obesity with only pharmacotherapy. Obesity medications are recommended for use only in cases with BMI $\geq$ 30 or BMI $\geq$ 27 with at least two risk factors. The NHLBI (1998a, 1998b) federal guidelines recommend that professionals prescribe a lifestyle behavioral approach for at least six months prior to attempting an obesity medication trial. Medications should be used as additional tools (i.e., as part of a comprehensive weight management program) to help selected patients achieve successful long-term weight management.

Lessons learned

These guidelines for pharmacotherapy are logical based on important lessons in the field. First, the seminal controlled treatment studies (Brownell & Stunkard, 1981; Craighead, 1984; Craighead, Stunkard, & O'Brien, 1981) as well as more recent controlled studies (Wadden, Berkowitz, Sarwer, Prus-Wisniewski, & Steinberg, 2001) have collectively found that adding behavior therapy to obesity medications enhances short and longer term outcomes but medications used alone are characterized by poorer outcomes than behavior therapy alone. Second, in the 1990s, two widely used and popular obesity medications – fenfluramine and dexfenfluramine – were removed from the market following a number of studies reporting major medical problems (i.e., primary pulmonary hypertension and heart valve abnormalities) associated with using these medications (Abenhaim et al., 1996; Kurz & Van Ermen, 1997; McCann et al., 1997). This so-called "phen-fen debacle" was further complicated with reports that many average weight persons were obtaining weight loss medications driven by cosmetic reasons. These incidents forced the field to confront serious challenges, including the need for longer trials to address safety and effectiveness. The federal guidelines (NHLBI, 1998a, 1998b) are now clear about when to consider obesity medications. The field now conceptualizes obesity as a chronic ongoing problem so any intervention (e.g., medication) must be considered in such a light.

Contraindications

Persons who meet the following criteria should not be treated with obesity medications: pregnant or lactating women; those with severe systemic illness or cardiac related conditions; those on other medication regimens that might adversely interact with the obesity medications (e.g., monoamine oxidase inhibitor antidepressants); and those with uncontrolled high blood pressure. Additional (less absolute) contraindications include: those under age 18 or over 65; history of certain severe mental illnesses (most notably psychosis, bipolar disorder, anorexia nervosa) and any current other severe mental disorders that might warrant more immediate attention (e.g., severe depression, anxiety, or substance use problems).

Obesity medications

At present, there are approximately ten FDA-approved medications for obesity in the United States, although several have abuse potential and are generally not recommended. Essentially, of those considered appropriate for use, there are two centrally active adrenergic medications (phentermine, diethylpropion), one centrally active combined adrenergic and serotenergic medication (sibutramine), and one locally active (orlistat). Only sibutramine and orlistat are currently approved for long-term use.

Adrenergic medications

These are only approved for short-term use and are now viewed as having little clinical role for treating obesity. Previous reviews of a large number of studies conducted with adrenergic medications conducted 20 years ago noted that in roughly 40% of the controlled treatment studies, medications produced significantly more weight loss than placebo. Across these short-term studies, the obesity medications averaged roughly one-half pound per week more weight loss (Bray, 1992). The most studied adrenergic drug is phentermine, which is still approved by the FDA for short-term treatment (i.e., three months or less). Phentermine recommended doses are 15 to 30 mg per day for the resin form and 18.75 to 37.5 mg per day for the hydrochloride form. Phentermine is associated with the following common side effects, which are experienced significantly more frequently than placebo: rapid heart beat, increased blood pressure, restlessness, constipation, and diminished sexual arousal.

Sibutramine

Sibutramine was approved by the FDA in 1997 as an obesity medication. Sibutramine is also currently approved for obesity in many countries worldwide (Centre for Pharmaceutical Administration, 2003; National Institute for Clinical Excellence (NICE), 2001/2004). Sibutramine is a centrally active serotonin and norepinephrine reuptake inhibitor (Arterburn, Crane, & Veenstra, 2004; Astrup, Hansen, Lundsgaard, & Toubro, 1998; Clapham, Arch, & Tadayyon, 2001). Numerous randomized placebo-controlled trials with diverse obese patient groups with and without medical co-morbidities performed in specialized and in generalist settings (e.g., Bray et al., 1999; Hanotin, Thomas, Jones, Leutenegger, & Drouin, 1998; Lean, 1997; Wirth & Krause, 2001) have reported sibutramine to be superior to placebo. Most research has been with doses of 10 mg to 20 mg once daily and most have reported similar efficacy and tolerability (side effects) for those doses (e.g., Hanotin et al., 1998). For obesity, it is frequently recommended that the starting dose be 10 mg/d and that dosing can be increased to 15 mg/d after several weeks (NICE 2001/2004).

Several studies have reported effectiveness and safety of sibutramine as used in primary care settings. The S.A.T. Study (Hauner et al., 2002), conducted with 389 obese patients at 33 general primary care practices, tested 15 mg/d of sibutramine versus placebo over a 54-week regimen. Sibutramine produced significantly greater weight loss than placebo (mean of 3.0 kg more) and was significantly more likely to achieve 5% weight loss than placebo (63% versus 41%). A modest increase in heart rate was reported for sibutramine. Almost identical results were reported by Smith and Goulder (2001) based on a study conducted with 485 patients with uncomplicated obesity also performed in primary care settings.

Several critical reviews have supported the efficacy of sibutramine for weight loss in obese patients (Centre for Pharmaceutical Administration, 2003; O'Meara, Riemsma, Shirran, Mather, & ter Riet, 2002). These reviews, however, have noted the need for careful medical monitoring of patients because of concerns for potential cardiovascular side effects (Centre for Pharmaceutical Administration, 2003; O'Meara et al., 2002). Arterburn and colleagues (2004) conducted the most recent systematic critical review of randomized placebo-controlled studies of sibutramine. Arterburn et al. (2004) selected 29 studies that were methodologically strong enough to be included in their meta-analysis. In three-month trials, the average difference in weight loss (sibutramine minus placebo) was -2.78 kg. In longer trials, this difference increased slightly over time, but so did dropout rates. Weight loss with sibutramine was associated with modest increases in blood pressure and heart rate. Although a number of published studies have reported safety data based on two years of sibutramine use, Arterburn et al. (2004) concluded that there is insufficient evidence to accurately determine the long-term risk–benefit profile for sibutramine. It is perhaps worth noting here that it appears that nearly all (if not all) of those studies were funded by the pharmaceutical companies.

There is consensus for the need for careful medical monitoring of patients taking sibutramine because of concerns for potential cardiovascular side effects (Centre for Pharmaceutical Administration, 2003; O'Meara et al., 2002). Reports indicate sibutramine increases heart rate and increases systolic and diastolic blood pressure roughly 2 mmHg in patients with normal blood pressure. Roughly 12% of patients experience clinically significant rises in blood pressure. Interestingly, in patients with hypertension, sibutramine seems to produce slight decreases in blood pressure. Other common side effects include mild degrees of dry mouth, constipation, and insomnia. Valvular heart disease has been observed in 2.3% of patients treated with sibutramine versus 2.6% of patients treated with placebo.

Orlistat

Orlistat, is a non-centrally acting medication approved as an anti-obesity medication by the FDA in 1999. Orlistat, a lipase inhibitor, works locally in the gut and inhibits digestion and absorption of dietary fat (Drent & Van der Veen, 1993). A maximum 30% reduction in fat absorption appears to be accomplished using a dose of 120 mg taken three times per day.

Studies have found that orlistat has efficacy for weight loss and for longer term weight control, i.e., over a two-year period (Davidson et al., 1999; Hauptman et al., 2000; O'Meara et al., 2004; Sjostrom et al., 1998). Davidson and colleagues (1999), in a large US study involving multiple sites, performed a double-blind placebo-controlled study. Patients treated with orlistat (120 mg three times daily) plus diet and behavior therapy lost significantly more weight (average of 5.8 kg more) than patients receiving placebo plus diet and behavior therapy during the first year of treatment. Use of higher dose of orlistat (120 mg three times daily) resulted in less weight regain (35% regain) than a lower dose (60 mg three times daily) and placebo (51% and 63% regain, respectively). The European Multicentre Orlistat Study Group (Sjostrom et al., 1998) reported similar weight loss/regain patterns. Both US (Davidson et al., 1999) and European (Sjostrom et al., 1998) studies reported that adding orlistat to diet was associated with significantly greater improvements than placebo in lipid profiles and insulin levels.

Orlistat has also received support for treating obese patients with type II diabetes in four controlled trials (Hanefeld & Sachse, 2002; Hollander et al., 1998; Kelley et al., 2002; Miles et al., 2002). These trials reported significant advantages for the orlistat over the placebo for weight losses (mean weight loss on orlistat ranged from −3.89 kg to −6.19 kg), likelihood of achieving 5% weight loss, and on most obesity-related outcomes (lipids).

Since orlistat works locally, not centrally, it does not have the same safety concerns that have existed for other obesity medications. Orlistat is, however, associated with common gastrointestinal side effects. Because considerable fat passes through the intestines, stool softening, oily stools and soiling, and increased stool size are common. Most treatment studies have found these side effects, while embarrassing, to be transient and to improve particularly as adjustments to eating are made. Since it is possible that important nutrients such as fat-soluble vitamins can be lost, persons taking orlistat should take vitamin supplements.

Sibutramine versus orlistat

Several studies have compared sibutramine and orlistat as well as their combination for treating obesity and associated co-morbidities.

Overall, these studies have generally provided additional support for the safety and effectiveness of these two medications. Some statistically significant differences emerged from these comparative studies. These differences, albeit modest from a clinical or effect size perspective, are as follows. Some studies have reported statistically superior weight losses for sibutramine versus orlistat (Gokcel et al., 2002; Kaya et al., 2004; Sari, Balci, Cakir, Altunbas, & Karayalcin, 2004) while others either failed to observe differences or found slight advantages for orlistat over sibutramine on some obesity measures (Derosa, Cicero, Murdolo, Ciccarelli, & Fogari, 2004; Derosa et al., 2005). One study found sibutramine produced greater reduction in both BMI and in waist circumference than orlistat (Gokcel et al., 2002) whereas other studies found that orlistat resulted in greater reduction in waist circumference than sibutramine (Aydin, Topsver, Kaya, Karasakal, Duman, & Dagar, 2004). A consistent finding is that the combination of sibutramine and orlistat is generally comparable to sibutramine alone but is superior to orlistat alone on most obesity variables (Aydin et al., 2004; Kaya et al., 2004; Sari et al., 2004).

What about obesity treatments for children and adolescents?

Childhood obesity, like adulthood obesity, has increased markedly during the past 20 years. As noted previously in chapter 2, estimates are that roughly 25% of children aged 6 to 11 years and adolescents aged 12 to 18 years are obese. Given the limitations in the effectiveness of treatments for obesity as described above, it seems critical that early intervention and treatments be given to children to improve health and well-being and to prevent them from becoming obese adults. The essential components for children and adolescents are the same as for adults. Weight control requires behavior change, improved coping, and sustainable changes in nutrition and physical activity necessary for energy balance. The obvious challenges include how to achieve this within appropriate developmental and maturational needs. These interventions also need to consider the family context (since parents provide and prepare foods) and preparation for handling multiple settings (school cafeterias, peer influences).

The most impressive interventions appear to be focused behavioral and family-based efforts (Epstein, Myers, Raynor, & Saelens, 1998). Much of these treatment methods were developed and tested by Epstein (Epstein, Wing, Koeske, & Valoski, 1985; Epstein et al., 1995). Impressive long-term outcomes have been documented for these behavioral family-based approaches (Epstein, Valoski, Wing, & McCurley, 1994). These family-based interventions rely on traditional behavior therapy principles and provide information and interventions tailored to the development needs of the children. For example, information on balanced nutrition follows the Food Guide Pyramid but is presented using a "terrific light" approach ("red light" for items to avoid based on high fat content ranging to "green light" for foods with low gram content per serving). Great care is taken to foster confidence and motivation to perform physical activity and to overcome the well-known preferences for sedentary activity (watching television, playing video games) in obese, poorly conditioned, and self-conscious youth. Parental modification of the food environment is a major focus. Parents are taught, encouraged, and asked to track their own progress in making changes to control the environment in terms of decreasing stimuli and availability of high fat unhealthy foods, increasing availability of healthy and tasty foods, increasing time and options for family physical activities, and for continued supportive interactions with the children. The importance of parental modeling is emphasized. These changes are beneficial for the entire family to follow. It is critical to view them as positive family changes rather than changes that are solely intended for the obese child. Thus, parents are expected to participate fully in these behavioral changes.

The potential role of obesity medications for younger patients is unknown. The FDA-approved obesity medications are only for use in adults but experimental research is beginning. Berkowitz, Wadden, Terschakovec, and Conquist (2003) recently performed the first randomized placebo-controlled study of sibutramine in obese adolescents (82 boys and girls aged 13 to 17 years). Berkowitz and colleagues (2003) reported that the addition of sibutramine to a comprehensive behavioral program resulted in greater weight loss than did the addition of placebo to the behavioral program. The authors emphasized that until more extensive safety and effectiveness data become available, medications for weight loss in adolescents should only be used within carefully controlled experimental studies. Such studies are underway.

Surgical interventions for obesity

Surgery for obesity will be described in greater detail than the previous interventions. This is for several reasons. First, outside the medical literature, surgery tends to be briefly or not at all noted.

Second, the past decade has seen a continued rise in extreme obesity and a marked increase in the use of surgery for obesity. Third, a large body of evidence has accumulated during the past decade supporting the use of surgery for obesity. The outcomes of surgery for obesity are striking in magnitude and scope and warrant careful discussion.

Surgical interventions for obesity date back to the 1950s (Deitel & Shikora, 2002; MacDonald, 2003) and can be divided into three broad categories. The three categories of surgical approaches include: (1) malabsorptive procedures, which interfere with digestion or absorption by altering the flow of food from the stomach to the intestine; (2) restrictive procedures, which reduce or limit the size of the stomach and how much food it can hold; (3) combination procedures, which involve a combination of both restrictive and malabsorption procedures.

The first surgeries for obesity involved malabsorption procedures. Clinical observations that persons with short-bowel syndrome lost weight led to attempting intestinal bypass procedures (jejuno-colic bypass) in 1954 and jejuno-ileal (JI) bypass from 1954 through the 1970s, when it became the standard method. JI bypass, which bypassed or excluded the majority of the small bowel (leaving less than 20 inches exposed to the passage of food), produced significant weight losses. This procedure was eventually banned due to the high rates of severe nutritional problems and nearly universal need for surgical reconnections.

The next major surgical approach involved refinements and extensions of restrictive procedures pioneered by Edward Mason at the University of Iowa Hospitals. For years, the primary surgeries involved various restrictive procedures, such as vertical banded gastroplasty and gastric banding which simply limited the stomach's capacity for food intake. These various restrictive procedures utilize various belts or devices placed on regions of the stomach to essentially make it smaller. The next major advance came after clinical observation of significant weight loss in a woman who underwent a partial gastrectomy for peptic ulcer. This led to the first gastric bypass surgery in 1967 described in the seminal paper by Mason and Ito (1967) and to the use of combining methods both to restrict food intake and to reduce absorption of food. Subsequent refinements (Griffin, Young, & Stevenson, 1977) lead to the Roux-en-Y gastric bypass (RYGB) method and variants led to current surgical approaches which are very successful and increasingly safe with fewer perioperative complications (Biertho et al., 2003; Buchwald & Buchwald, 2002; MacDonald, 2003).

Today, most surgeries for obesity (now termed bariatric surgery) involve combination procedures, such as RYGB gastric bypass, which tend to maximize weight loss. The two other major types of combined procedures are the biliopancreatic diversion (Scopinario procedure) and a modification known as the duodenal switch procedure. Although both of these diversion methods appear to produce even greater weight losses than the gastric bypass methods, they are associated with higher rates of serious complications. Readers interested in descriptions of these and other current bariatric surgical procedures and how they evolved from the initial methods started in the 1950s are referred to Buchwald and Buchwald (2002) and Deitel and Shikora (2002).

Perhaps the major development in the past decade has been the use of laparoscopic surgery. Through the use of specialized instruments, including the laparoscope sending images to a TV monitor, these surgeries have become significantly less invasive. Laparoscopic approaches have, for many patients, eliminated the need for large abdominal incisions and have allowed for the surgery to be performed in a minimally invasive manner. Laparoscopic bariatric surgeries have resulted in much faster postoperative recovery, healing, and return to regular activities (Cottam, Nguyen, Eid, & Schauer, 2005; Wittgrove & Clark, 2000).

The past decades have witnessed a rapid increase in bariatric surgery. The annual rate of bariatric surgery in the United States more than doubled from 1990 to 1997 (Pope, Birkmeyer, & Finlayson, 2002). Recent years have seen a further escalation in the use of these surgeries in the US and worldwide (Buchwald & Williams, 2004). Rates of bariatric surgeries were estimated to increase from 28,000 surgeries in 2000 to 120,000 surgeries in 2003 (Mitka, 2003).

Bariatric surgery outcomes

Overall, studies generally report weight losses of roughly 40% of excess weight within six months of surgery with the maximum weight loss (roughly 50–60%) generally achieved by two years after surgery. In striking contrast to all other obesity treatments and weight loss methods, the weight loss produced by bariatric surgery is both substantial and highly durable over time. Studies have reported average weight losses of roughly 50% successfully maintained in long-term follow-up studies conducted five to ten years after surgery. Particularly impressive are the consistent findings across many studies worldwide that a very substantial majority of severely obese patients have marked or full resolution in serious obesity-related co-morbidities, including diabetes, hyperlipidemia, and hypertension (Schauer et al., 2003; Sjostrom, Lissner, Wedel, & Sjostrom, 1999; Sugarman, Wolfe, Sica, & Clore, 2003b). Bariatric surgery, in addition to the important health improvements, is also economically cost effective. Sampalis, Liberman, Auger, and Christou (2004) demonstrated that the costs of bariatric surgery are amortized within about 3.5 years. Thus, in addition to effective weight loss, very substantial decreases occur in long-term health care costs by severely obese patients who undergo bariatric surgery (Sampalis et al., 2004). Another recent analysis documented significant decreases in long-term mortality by severely obese patients who underwent bariatric surgery in addition to long-term decreases in morbidity and in health care use (Christou et al., 2004).

A systematic review and meta-analysis conducted by Buchwald and colleagues (2004) summarized the empirical evidence from 136 bariatric surgery studies comprising a total of 22,094 patients. The mean excess weight loss across all of these studies was 61.2%. Mean weight losses were greater for the combined procedures such as gastric bypass (68.2%) than for purely restrictive methods such as gastric banding. Diabetes was completely resolved in 76.8% of patients, hypertension was completely resolved in 61.7% of patients, and obstructive sleep apnea was resolved in 85.7% of patients. In terms of improvements in the medical co-morbidities, while the major surgical approaches were all generally effective, there were some important differences across different surgical techniques. In particular, complete resolution of diabetes was observed as follows: 98.9% (for biliopancreatic diversion or duodenal switch), 83.7% (for gastric bypass), 71.6% (for gastroplasty), and 47.9% (for gastric banding).

These improvements in associated metabolic and medical problems in extremely obese patients following bariatric surgery are truly impressive. The nearly universal resolution of diabetes, for example, is in sharp contrast to the well-known challenges and difficulties in managing that problem with state-of-the-art medications and behavioral therapies. In addition to representing a potential method for wider use for medical conditions such as type II diabetes (Pories et al., 1995), bariatric surgery has served as a vehicle for improving our understanding of the pathophysiology of metabolic disturbances. For example, the effect of gastric bypass surgery on the metabolic syndrome and diabetes is likely due to the bypass of the hormonally active foregut, rather than from weight loss per se. The normalization of glucose tolerance in these patients is remarkably rapid, frequently occurring within ten days of surgery, before any significant weight loss has occurred (Hickey et al., 1998; Pories et al., 1995). In contrast to the outcomes for diabetes, although hypertension improves dramatically during the year following bariatric surgery, longer follow-up studies have observed some return of hypertension in subsequent years (Sjostrom et al., 1999, Sjostrom, Peltonen, Wedel, & Sjostrom, 2000).

Roux-en-Y gastric bypass

Overall, Roux-en-Y gastric bypass (RYGB) produces more weight loss and greater medical improvements compared to other surgical procedures with fewer complications (Biertho et al., 2003; Buchwald et al., 2004; Sjostrom et al., 2004) and the weight loss is extremely well maintained over the long term. The Roux-en-Y gastric bypass (RYGB) method is currently generally regarded as the "gold standard" given its impressive clinical outcomes (weight loss plus broad improvements in co-morbidities) coupled with good safety record. A recent international study of bariatric surgeries reported that laparoscopic gastric bypass was the most frequently used method (Buchwald & Williams, 2004). RYGB involves the surgical creation of a 15–50 mL gastric pouch, transecting the jejunum, and attaching the transected jejunum to the surgically created stomach pouch (see Figure 6.4).

Psychosocial and behavioral predictors and outcomes

The majority of studies investigating bariatric surgery outcomes have focused on postoperative weight loss and medical co-morbidities as the primary outcome. The high rates of psychological (e.g., depression, severe body image distress) and behavioral problems (e.g., binge eating problems) in bariatric surgery candidates (Elder et al., 2006; Grilo et al., 2005a) led naturally to concerns about selection and psychosocial criteria (Herpertz, Kielmann, Wolf, Hebebrand, & Senf, 2004). Herpertz and colleagues (2004) in their review of psychosocial factors of bariatric surgery outcomes concluded that preoperative psychiatric status, psychological functioning, personality and psychosocial functioning had surprisingly little predictive value for bariatric surgery outcomes. These findings continue to be supported across diverse bariatric surgery patients (Grilo et al., 2006; Latner, Wetzler, Goodman, & Glinski, 2004).

Research studies conducted with bariatric surgery patients have found that many of the psychological and behavioral problems seem to improve dramatically along with the substantial weight losses and

Figure 6.4.

Gastric bypass
(Roux-en-Y).

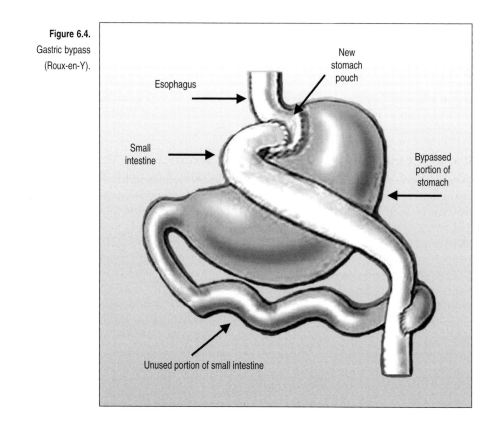

Esophagus

New stomach pouch

Small intestine

Bypassed portion of stomach

Unused portion of small intestine

robust improvements in medical co-morbidities. Herpertz, Kielmann, Wolf, Langkafel, Senf, & Hebebrand (2003) reviewed 40 studies with a minimum of one-year postoperative follow-up on psychosocial functioning following surgery. These studies consistently found that bariatric surgery, in addition to the substantial weight loss, is associated with decreased psychological distress, reduced anxiety and depressive symptoms, improved body image, and improved social and occupational functioning. These empirical findings challenge widespread beliefs that such psychological factors should automatically represent contraindications for surgery (Latner et al., 2004).

Swedish Obese Subjects Study

The interested reader is referred specifically to the prospective controlled Swedish Obese Subjects (SOS) Study (Sjostrom et al., 2004). This landmark controlled study is remarkable in terms of size, scope, and methodology, has produced particularly convincing ten-year outcome data across weight loss, medical co-morbidities and health indicators, broad psychosocial functioning, and economic domains supporting the superior effectiveness of bariatric surgery compared to non-surgical interventions (Sjostrom et al., 2004).

Adverse outcomes

Bariatric surgeries are major procedures with associated risks. The past 20 years have witnessed significant advances in these surgical methods. Today, they are generally considered to be safe when performed by appropriately trained surgeons and when performed following established guidelines. Good compliance by patients with nutritional and dietary guidelines postoperatively decreases the risks for complications. The rate of mortality immediately following surgery (within one month) is about 0.1% from purely restrictive surgeries, 0.5% from gastric bypass procedures, and as high as about 1.1% from bibliopancreatic diversion or duodenal switch procedures (Buchwald et al., 2004).

This is not to say that adverse events are not common. The rates of adverse events and complications differ somewhat across the different types of bariatric surgeries. Surgeries that rely primarily on restrictive methods have higher rates of ruptures while those that capitalize on malabsorption have higher rates of nutritional consequences. In general, common risks include bleeding, infections, gallstones (due to rapid weight loss), and inflammation of the stomach lining. Nutritional complications can occur, particularly if patients do not follow nutritional and dietary guidelines. The most common nutritional complications include dehydration, vitamin (i.e., B12) and iron deficiencies (which can result in anemia), and calcium deficiency (which can contribute to bone problems). Follow-up surgeries to correct these complications (as well as to remove excess skin) are not uncommon, although the recent use of laparoscopic methods appears to have decreased the need for additional surgeries to some degree.

Immediately following the surgeries, physical pain and discomfort are universal and, like most major surgeries, not insignificant. Laparoscopic methods have reduced these physical sequelae substantially (Cottam et al., 2005). The patient must then learn to eat in small quantities and to chew the food completely. The patients must learn to do this gradually to transition successfully from puréed foods as the small stomach pouch expands slightly. Risk for dehydration is high immediately after and for several months following bariatric surgeries. Many patients have difficulty drinking enough liquid as they struggle to adapt to the much smaller stomach capacity.

A common complication following gastric bypass and other bariatric surgeries is "dumping syndrome." Symptoms include nausea and vomiting, diarrhea, bloating, dizziness, and bouts of sweating. It is critical, especially during the first few months following the surgery, to follow specific dietary guidelines to decrease these symptoms and to decrease the chances of other complications.

These risks must be considered carefully by any prospective patient. The surgical risks must be considered against standards. First, the patient must consider the existing heightened risk for morbidity and mortality associated with the severe obesity (i.e., not losing the weight poses high risk). Second, the patient must consider the risk against the very high likelihood of benefits associated with the surgery.

Bariatric surgery guidelines

The 1992 NIH Consensus Conference on Gastrointestinal Surgery for Severe Obesity established guidelines for surgical treatment of morbid obesity in the United States. This panel of experts concluded that the rationale for surgery for obesity was based on consistent findings from many studies indicating that standard treatments for obesity (dietary weight reduction with or without behavior therapy or pharmacotherapy) had unacceptably high rates of weight regain in severely obese persons within two years after losing weight. The NIH guidelines specified that severely obese adults could be eligible for bariatric surgery for obesity if they have a BMI greater than 40 or a BMI greater than 35 if an obesity-related medical problem is present.

What about bariatric surgery for severely obese adolescents?

Of note is that the NIH guidelines for bariatric surgery pertain to adults. This raises the important issue about whether to consider bariatric surgery in adolescents who are severely obese and are already suffering from associated medical problems. There were few available studies on bariatric surgery in obese adolescents (Anderson, Soper, & Scott, 1980) when the NIH guidelines were published in 1991. Since then, several studies have addressed the clinical and safety issues of bariatric surgery in adolescents and whether such interventions are warranted (Greenstein & Rabner, 1995; Rand & MacGregor, 1994; Strauss, Bradley, & Brolin, 2001; Sugarman et al., 2003a). Except for the early 1980 report (Anderson et al., 1980) which included several cases with severe mental retardation and two operative deaths, there were no reported postoperative deaths in the adolescents in the more recent studies. Sugarman and his colleagues (2003a) reported significant and long-lasting weight losses, resolution or significant improvement in most medical co-morbidities, and substantial improvements in psychosocial functioning in their adolescent bariatric surgery cases. The clinical outcomes and safety data were generally consistent with those found in the research literature for severely obese adults who undergo bariatric surgery.

Bariatric surgery is still rarely performed in adolescents (e.g., less than 1% of the total surgeries performed by the Sugarman group in over 20 years (Sugarman et al., 2003a)), although it is probably increasing, along with the figures for adults (Mitka, 2003). The recent increase in severe obesity in younger persons highlights the need for continued investigation of whether to lower the age for bariatric surgery. Kral and colleagues (2002), and others (Apovian et al., 2005), highlighted the need for further discussion and research on the role of bariatric surgery at younger ages given uncertainties about potential long-term problems and uncertainty about the safety of future pregnancies.

Summary

Obesity is now viewed as one of the major public health problems in the world. It is increasingly recognized as a serious medical condition rather than as a reflection of "lack of willpower." Although much hope and excitement now exists in the scientific community around remarkable advances in molecular genetics and mapping the human obesity gene (Perusse et al., 2005), the exact causes of obesity remain uncertain. It is increasingly evident that major public health and massive environmental shifts are needed to interrupt the current trend of a continued increase in obesity. Finding ways to promote eating less (smaller portions), eating less fat, avoiding empty calories (soft drinks), and increasing lifestyle and recreational physical activity levels are pressing issues. It is critical to find ways to begin achieving these changes during childhood before obesity and unhealthy behaviors become entrenched. The challenge is to develop and foster environments in families, communities, and schools that facilitate healthy behaviors (healthy eating, healthy body image, and healthy exercise) while taking care to avoid harsh or critical messages that promote eating concerns or disorders. Clinically, in the case of persons already suffering from obesity, compassion and respect must not be overlooked when attempting to work with this challenging problem. The major question facing obesity treatment and research remains how to best facilitate successful long-term weight maintenance. Diverse approaches promote weight loss, but except for the special case of bariatric surgery for severely obese patients, most approaches are characterized by weight regain in subsequent years.

Further reading and resources

There are many additional resources available for the interested reader. This book has used a relatively heavy citation and referencing approach. This approach reflects the author's strong bias to rely, wherever possible, on empirical research. This book was not intended to be comprehensive in its coverage of the topic areas. Instead, the goal was to provide a balanced authoritative overview of the eating and weight disorders along with a reasonably representative list of the major references for the main points and conclusions.

The remarkable access to information by the world-wide-web represents a major resource. Information is readily available. There is also a significant downside. In the case of eating disorders and obesity, there is a staggering amount of information available that unfortunately ranges from incorrect to harmful and dangerous. In the case of obesity, there is widespread advertising of "miracle" diets and weight loss products that desperate persons repeatedly fall prey to. In the case of anorexia nervosa, there are websites and so-called "chat rooms" that foster and encourage dangerous extreme weight loss methods. With this context in mind, a very few select organizations are listed below that provide information that is balanced and consistent with our (still limited) body of knowledge.

Each of these organizations includes links to additional resources. Each of these organizations has information specifically geared to the public, students, professional, patients, and family members and lists education and training opportunities for all levels of interested parties.

- National Institutes of Health in the United States
- National Institute for Clinical Excellence in the United Kingdom
- Academy for Eating Disorders
- North American Association for the Study of Obesity.

Treatment manuals

Specific treatment manuals have been referenced throughout the text. A fair amount of attention was devoted to specific self-help methods that have received some support from controlled research. The titles listed in the box below include several self-help programs written specifically for clients. These programs were selectively chosen from a fairly large number of such publications available on the market. These specific manuals were written by recognized experts in their respective fields. In addition, each of these manuals has received some scrutiny in research settings.

SELF-HELP PROGRAMS FOR EATING AND WEIGHT DISORDERS WITH EMPIRICAL SUPPORT

Eating disorders

Apple, R. F., & Agras, W. S. (1997). *Client workbook: Overcoming binge eating: A cognitive-behavioral treatment for bulimia nervosa and binge eating disorder.* San Antonio: Psychological Corporation and Graywind Publications.
Cooper, P. J. (1995). *Bulimia nervosa and binge eating: A guide to recovery.* London: Robinson.
Fairburn, C. G. (1995). *Overcoming binge eating.* New York: Guilford Press.
Schmidt, U. H., & Treasure, J. L. (1993). *Getting better bit(e) by bit(e).* Hove, UK: Lawrence Erlbaum Associates Ltd.

For parents of children and adolescents with eating disorders

Bryant-Waugh, R. J., & Lask, B. (2004). *Eating disorders: A parents' guide.* London: Brunner-Routledge.
Walsh, B. T., & Cameron, V. L. (2005). *If your adolescent has an eating disorder.* New York: Oxford University Press.

Obesity and weight control

Blair, S. N. (1991). *Living with exercise: Improving your health through moderate physical activity.* Dallas, TX: American Health Publishing.
Brownell, K. D. (2000). *The LEARN program for weight management.* Dallas, TX: American Health Publishing.

Related problems

Cash, T. F. (1997). *The body image workbook: An 8-step program for learning to like your looks.* Oakland, CA: New Harbinger Publications.

Note: Expanded adaptation based on Grilo (2000) review of research on self-help approaches for eating and weight disorders.

References

Abenhaim, L., Moride Y., Brenot F., Rich, S., Benichou, J., Kurz, X., et al. (1996). Appetite-suppressant drugs and the risk of primary pulmonary hypertension: International Primary Pulmonary Hypertension Study Group. *New England Journal of Medicine, 335,* 606–666.

Abraham, S. F., & Beumont, P. J. (1982). How patients describe bulimia or binge eating. *Psychological Medicine, 12,* 625–635.

Ackard, D. M., Neumark-Sztainer, D., Story, M., & Perry, C. (2003). Overeating among adolescents: Prevalence and associations with weight-related characteristics and psychological health. *Pediatrics, 111,* 67–74.

Agras, W. S. (1997). Pharmacotherapy of bulimia nervosa and binge eating disorder: Longer-term outcomes. *Psychopharmacology Bulletin, 33,* 433–436.

Agras, W. S., Barlow, D. H., Chapin, H. N., Abel, G. G., & Leitenberg, H. (1974). Behavior modification of anorexia nervosa. *Archives of General Psychiatry, 30,* 279, 286.

Agras, W. S., Brandt, H. A., Bulik, C. M., Dolan-Sewell, R., Fairburn, C. G., Halmi, K. A., et al. (2004). Report of the National Institutes of Health workshop on overcoming barriers to treatment research in anorexia nervosa. *International Journal of Eating Disorders, 35,* 509–521.

Agras, W. S., Crow, S. J., Halmi, K. A., Mitchell, J. E., Wilson, G. T., & Kraemer, H. C. (2000a). Outcome predictors for the cognitive behavioral treatment of bulimia nervosa: Data from a multisite study. *American Journal of Psychiatry, 157,* 1302–1308.

Agras, W. S., & Kraemer, H. C. (1983). The treatment of anorexia nervosa: Do different treatments have different outcomes? *Psychiatric Annals, 13,* 928–935.

Agras, W. S., Rossiter, E. M., Arnow, B., Schneider, J. A., Telch, C. F., Raeburn, S. D., et al. (1992). Pharmacologic and cognitive-behavioral treatment for bulimia nervosa: A controlled comparison. *American Journal of Psychiatry, 149,* 82–87.

Agras, W. S., Telch, C. F., Arnow, B., Eldredge, K., & Marnell, M. (1997). One-year follow-up of cognitive behavioral therapy for obese individuals with binge eating disorder. *Journal of Consulting and Clinical Psychology, 65,* 343–347.

Agras, W. S., Telch, C. F., Arnow, B., Eldredge, K., Wilfley, D. E., Raeburn, S. D., et al. (1994). Weight loss, cognitive-behavioral, and desipramine treatments in binge eating disorder: An additive design. *Behavior Therapy, 25,* 225–238.

Agras, W. S., Walsh, B. T., Fairburn, C. G.,

Wilson, G. T., & Kraemer, H. C. (2000b). A multicenter comparison of cognitive-behavioral therapy and interpersonal psychotherapy for bulimia nervosa. *Archives of General Psychiatry, 57,* 459–466.

Akan, G. E., & Grilo, C. M. (1995). Sociocultural influences on eating attitudes and behaviors, body image, and psychological functioning: A comparison of African-American, Asian-American, and Caucasian college women. *International Journal of Eating Disorders, 18,* 181–187.

Alger, S. A., Schwalberg, M. D., Bigaouette, J. M., Michalek, A. V., & Howard, L. J. (1991). Effect of a tricyclic antidepressant and opiate antagonist on binge-eating behavior in normal weight bulimic and obese binge-eating subjects. *American Journal of Clinical Nutrition, 53,* 865–871.

Allison, D. B., Fontaine, K. R., Manson, J. E., Stevens, J., & VanItallie, T. B. (1999). Annual deaths attributable to obesity in the United States. *Journal of the American Medical Association, 282,* 1530–1538.

Allison, K. C., Grilo, C. M., Masheb, R. M., & Stunkard, A. J. (2005). Binge eating disorder and night eating syndrome: A comparative study of disordered eating. *Journal of Consulting and Clinical Psychology, 73,* 1107–1115.

American Diabetes Association (ADA) Expert Committee (2004). Diagnosis and classification of diabetes mellitus. *Diabetes Care, 27,* S5–S10.

American Diabetes Association (ADA) (2004). Screening for type 2 diabetes. *Diabetes Care, 27,* S11–S14.

American Psychiatric Association. (1994). *Diagnostic and statistical manual of mental disorders* (4th ed.). Washington, DC: American Psychiatric Association Press.

American Psychiatric Association. (2000a). *Diagnostic and statistical manual of mental disorders* (4th ed., text revision). Washington, DC: American Psychiatric Association Press.

American Psychiatric Association. (2000b). Practice guidelines for the treatment of patients with eating disorders (revision). *American Journal of Psychiatry, 157,* 1–39.

Anderluh, M. B., Tchanturia, K., Rabe-Hesketh, S., et al. (2003). Childhood obsessive-compulsive personality traits in adult women with eating disorders: Defining a broader eating disorder phenotype. *American Journal of Psychiatry, 160,* 242–247.

Anderluh, M. B., Tchanturia, K., Rabe-Hesketh, S., & Treasure, J. (2003). Childhood obsessive-compulsive personality traits in adult women with eating disorders: Defining a broader eating disorder phenotype. *American Journal of Psychiatry, 160,* 242–247.

Andersen, A., Bowers, W., & Evans, K. (1997). Inpatient treatment of anorexia nervosa. In D. Garner & P. Garfinkel (Eds.), *Handbook of treatment for eating disorders,* (2nd ed., pp. 327–353). New York: Guilford Press.

Andersen, A., & Holman, J. E. (1997). Males with eating disorders: Challenges for treatment and research. *Psychopharmacological Bulletin, 33,* 391–397.

Andersen, R. E., Wadden, T. A., Bartlett, S. J., Zemel, B., Verde, T. J., & Franckowiak, S. C. (1999). Lifestyle activity versus structured aerobic exercise to change body composition and cardiovascular risk factors in obese women: A randomized trial. *Journal of the American Medical Association, 281,* 335–340.

Anderson, A. E., Soper, R. T., & Scott, D. H. (1980). Gastric bypass for morbid obesity in children and adolescents. *Journal of Pediatric Surgery, 15,* 876–881.

Anderson, C., Peterson, C. B., Fletcher, L., Mitchell, J. E., Thuras, P., & Crow, S. J. (2001). Weight loss and gender: An examination of physician attitudes. *Obesity Research, 9,* 257–263.

Anderson, J. W., Brinkman-Kaplan, V., Hamilton, C. C., Logan, J. E., Collins, R. W., & Gustafson, N. J. (1994). Food-containing hypocaloric diets are as effective as liquid-supplement diets for obese individuals with NIDDM. *Diabetes Care, 17,* 602–604.

Apovian, C. M., Baker, C., Ludwig, D. S., Hoppin, A. G., Hsu, G., Lenders, C., et al. (2005). Best practice guidelines in pediatric/adolescent weight loss surgery. *Obesity Research, 13,* 274–282.

Appelbaum, P. S., & Rumpf, T. (1998). Civil commitment of the anorexic patient. *General Hospital Psychiatry, 20,* 225–230.

Appolinario, J. C., Bacaltchuk, J., Sichieri, R., Claudino, A. M., Gody-Matos, A., Morgan, C., et al. (2003). A randomized double-blind placebo-controlled study of sibutramine in the treatment of binge eating disorder. *Archives of General Psychiatry, 60,* 1109–1116.

Arnold, L. M., McElroy, S. L., Hudson, J. I., Welge, J. A., Bennett, A. J., & Keck, P. E. (2002). A placebo-controlled randomized trial of fluoxetine in the treatment of binge eating disorder. *Journal of Clinical Psychiatry, 63,* 1028–1033.

Arterburn, D. E., Crane, P. K., & Veenstra, D. L. (2004). The efficacy and safety of sibutramine for weight loss: A systematic review. *Archives of Internal Medicine, 164,* 994–1003.

Asbeck, I., Mast, M., Bierwag, A., Westenhofer, J., Acheson, K. J., & Muller, M. J. (2002). Severe underreporting of energy intake in normal weight subjects: Use of an appropriate standard and relation to restrained eating. *Public Health and Nutrition, 5,* 683–690.

Astrup, A. (2005). Super-sized and diabetic by frequent fast-food consumption? *Lancet, 365,* 4–5.

Astrup, A., Hansen, D. L., Lundsgaard, C., & Toubro, S. (1998). Sibutramine and energy balance. *International Journal of Obesity and Related Metabolic Disorders, 22,* 30–35.

Attia, E., Haiman, C., Walsh, B. T., & Flater, S. R. (1998). Does fluoxetine augment the inpatient treatment of anorexia nervosa? *American Journal of Psychiatry, 155,* 548–551.

Aydin, N., Topsver, P., Kaya, A., Karasakal, M., Duman, C., & Dagar, A. (2004). Orlistat, sibutramine, or combination, therapy: Which performs better on waist circumference in relation with body mass index in obese patients? *Tohoku Journal of Experimental Medicine, 202,* 173–180.

Bacaltchuk, J., & Hay, P. J. (2003). Antidepressants versus placebo for bulimia nervosa. *Cochrane Database Systematic Reviews 4,* CD003391.

Bachrach, L. K., Guido, D., Katzman, D., Litt, I. F., & Marcus, R. (1990). Decreased bone density in adolescent girls with anorexia nervosa. *Pediatrics, 86,* 440–447.

Bachrach, L. K., Katzman, D. K., Litt, I. F., Guido, D., & Marcus, R. (1991). Recovery from osteopenia in adolescent girls with anorexia nervosa. *Journal of Endocrinology and Metabolism, 72,* 602–606.

Bailer, U., de Zwaan, M., Leisch, F., Strnad, A., Lennkh-Wolfsberg, C., El-Giamal, N., et al. (2004). Guided self-help versus cognitive-behavioral group therapy in the treatment of bulimia nervosa. *International Journal of Eating Disorders, 35,* 522–537.

Banting, W. (1993). Letter on corpulence addressed to the public, 3rd edition. *Obesity Research, 1,* 153–163.

Baran, S. A., Weltzin, T. E., & Kaye, W. H. (1995). Low discharge weight and outcome in anorexia nervosa. *American Journal of Psychiatry, 152,* 1070–1072.

Barlow, C. E., Kohl, H. W., Gibbons, L. W.,

& Blair, S. N. (1995). Physical fitness, mortality and obesity. *International Journal of Obesity, 19*, S41–S44.

Barry, D. T., & Grilo, C. M. (2002). Eating and body image disturbances in adolescent psychiatric inpatients: Gender and ethnicity patterns. *International Journal of Eating Disorders, 32*, 335–343.

Barry, D. T., Grilo, C. M., & Masheb, R. M. (2002). Gender differences in patients with binge eating disorder. *International Journal of Eating Disorders, 31*, 63–70.

Barry, D. T., Grilo C. M., & Masheb, R. M. (2003). Comparison of patients with bulimia nervosa, obese patients with binge eating disorder, and nonobese patients with binge eating disorder. *Journal of Nervous and Mental Disorders, 191*, 589–594.

Baum, C. L., & Ford, W. F. (2004). The wage effects of obesity: A longitudinal study. *Health Economics, 13*, 885–899.

Beale, B., McMaster, R., & Hillege, S. (2004–2005). Eating disorders: A qualitative analysis of the parents' journey. *Contemporary Nurse, 18*, 124–132.

Becker, A. E., Keel, P., Anderson-Fye, E. P., & Thomas, J. J. (2004). Genes and/or jeans?: Genetic and socio-cultural contributions to risk for eating disorders. *Journal of Addictive Disorders, 23*, 81–103.

Ben-Tovim, D. I., Walker, K., Gilchrist, P., Freeman, R., Kalucy, R., & Esterman, A. (2001). Outcome in patients with eating disorders: A 5-year study. *Lancet, 357*, 1254–1257.

Berglas, S., & Levendusky, P. G. (1985). The therapeutic contract program: An individual-oriented psychological treatment community. *Psychotherapy: Theory, Research, Practice, Training, 22*, 36–45.

Berkowitz, R. I., Wadden, T. A., Tershakovec, A. M., & Conquist, J. L. (2003). Behavior therapy and sibutramine for the treatment of adolescent obesity: A randomized controlled trial. *Journal of the American Medical Association, 289*, 1805–1812.

Berscheid, E., Walster, E., & Bohrnstedt, G. (1973). The happy American body: A survey report. *Psychology Today, 7*, 119–131.

Beumont, P. J., Russell, J. D., & Touyz, S. W. (1993). Treatment of anorexia nervosa. *Lancet, 341*, 1635–1640.

Biederman, J., Herzog, D. B., Rivinus, T. M., Harper, G. P., Ferber, R. A., Rosenbaum, J. F., et al. (1985). Amitriptyline in the treatment of anorexia nervosa: A double-blind, placebo-controlled study. *Journal of Clinical Psychopharmacology, 5*, 10–16.

Biertho, L., Steffen, R., Ricklin, T., Horber, F. F., Pomp, A., Inabnet, W. B., et al. (2003). Laparoscopic gastric bypass versus laparoscopic adjustable gastric banding: A comparative study of 1,200 cases. *Journal of the American College of Surgeons, 197*, 536–545.

Binford, R. B., Le Grange, D., & Jellar, C. C. (2004). Eating Disorders Examination versus Eating Disorders Examination-Questionnaire in adolescents with full and partial syndrome bulimia nervosa and anorexia nervosa. *International Journal of Eating Disorders, 37*, 44–49.

Birketvedt, G. S., Florholmen, J., Sundsfjord, J., Osterud, B., Dinges, D., Bilker, W., et al. (1999). Behavioral and neuroendocrine characteristics of the night eating syndrome. *Journal of the American Medical Association, 282*, 657–663.

Birmingham, C. L., Su, J., Hlynsky, J. A., Goldner, E. M., & Gao, M. (2005). The mortality rate from anorexia nervosa. *International Journal of Eating Disorders, 38*, 143–146.

Bish, C. L., Blanck, H. M., Serdula, M. K., Marcus, M., Kohl, H. W., & Khan, L. K. (2005). Diet and physical activity behaviors among Americans trying to lose weight: 2000 Behavioral Risk Factor Surveillance System. *Obesity Research, 13*, 596–607.

Black, C. M., & Wilson, G. T. (1996). Assessment of eating disorders: Interview versus questionnaire. *International Journal of Eating Disorders, 20*, 43–59.

Blackburn, G. (1995). Effect of degree of weight loss on health benefits. *Obesity Research, 3*, 211S–216S.

Blackburn, G. (1999). Benefits of weight loss in the treatment of obesity. *American Journal of Clinical Nutrition, 69*, 347–349.

Bonnet, M. H., & Arand, D. L. (1995). We are chronically sleep-deprived. *Sleep, 18*, 908–911.

Bowman, S. A., Gortmaker, S. L., Ebbeling, C. B., Pereira, M. A., & Ludwig, D. S. (2004). Effects of fast-food consumption on energy intake and diet quality among children in a national household survey. *Pediatrics, 113*, 112–118.

Braun, D. L., Sunday, S. R., & Halmi, K. A. (1994). Psychiatric comorbidity in patients with eating disorders. *Psychological Medicine, 24*, 859–867.

Bray, G. A. (1992). Drug treatment of obesity. *American Journal of Clinical Nutrition, 55*, 538–544.

Bray, G. A. (1993). Commentary on classics in obesity: Science and politics of hunger. *Obesity Research, 1*, 489–493.

Bray, G. A. (2002a). Predicting obesity in adults from childhood and adolescent weight. *American Journal of Clinical Nutrition, 76*, 497–498.

Bray, G. A. (2002b). A brief history of obesity. In C. G. Fairburn & K. D. Brownell (Eds.), *A comprehensive handbook of eating disorders and obesity* (2nd ed., pp. 382–387). New York: Guilford Press.

Bray, G. A., Blackburn, G. L., Ferguson, J. M., Greenway, F. L, Jain, A. K., Mendel, C. M., et al. (1999). Sibutramine produces dose-related weight loss. *Obesity Research, 7*, 189–198.

Bray, G. A., & Champagne, C. M. (2005). Beyond energy balance: There is more to obesity than kilocalories. *Journal of the American Dietetic Association, 105*, 17–23.

Bray, G. A., Nielsen, S. J., & Popkin, B. M. (2004). Consumption of high-fructose corn syrup in beverages may play a role in the epidemic of obesity. *American Journal of Clinical Nutrition, 79*, 537–543.

Bray, G. A., & Popkin, B. M. (1998). Dietary fat intake does affect obesity! *American Journal of Clinical Nutrition, 68*, 1157–1173.

Bray, G. A., & Popkin, B. M. (1999). Dietary fat affects obesity rate. *American Journal of Clinical Nutrition, 70*, 572–573.

Brener, N. D., Grunbaum, J. A., Kann, L., McManus, T., & Ross, J. (2004). Assessing health risk behaviors among adolescents: The effect of question wording and appeals for honesty. *Journal of Adolescent Health, 35*, 91–100.

Brewerton, T. D., Lydiard, R. B., Herzog, D. B., Brotman, A. W., O'Neil, P. M., & Ballenger, J. C. (1995a). Comorbidity of axis I psychiatric disorders in bulimia nervosa. *Journal of Clinical Psychiatry, 56*, 77–80.

Brewerton, T. D., Stellefson, E. J., Hibbs, N., Hodges, E. L., & Cochrane, C. E. (1995b). Comparison of eating disorder patients with and without compulsive exercising. *International Journal of Eating Disorders, 17*, 413–416.

Brody, M. L., Walsh, B. T., & Devlin, M. J. (1994). Binge eating disorder: Reliability and validity of a new diagnostic category. *Journal of Consulting and Clinical Psychology, 62*, 381–386.

Brownell, K. D. (2000). *LEARN 2000 Program For Weight Control*. Dallas, TX: American Health Publishing.

Brownell, K. D., & Jeffery, R. W. (1987). Improving long-term weight loss: Pushing the limits of treatment. *Behavior Therapy, 18*, 353–374.

Brownell, K. D., & Napolitano, M. A. (1995). Distorting reality for children: Body size proportions of Barbie and Ken dolls. *International Journal of Eating Disorders, 18*, 295–298.

Brownell, K., & Rodin, J. (1994). Medical, metabolic, and psychological effects of weight cycling. *Archives of Internal Medicine, 154*, 1325–1330.

Brownell, K. D., & Stunkard, A. J. (1981). Couples training, pharmocotherapy, and behavior therapy in the treatment of obesity. *Archives of General Psychiatry, 38*, 1224–1229.

Brownell, K. D., & Wadden, T. A. (1991). The heterogeneity of obesity: Fitting treatments to the individual. *Behavior Therapy, 22*, 153–177.

Brownell K., & Wadden, T. A. (1992). Etiology and treatment of obesity: Understanding a serious, prevalent, and refractory disorder. *Journal of Consulting and Clinical Psychology, 60*, 505–517.

Browning, R. C., & Kram, R. (2005). Energetic cost and preferred speed of walking in obese vs. normal weight women. *Obesity Research, 13*, 891–899.

Bryant-Waugh, R. J., Cooper, P. J., Taylor, C. L., & Lask, B. D. (1996). The use of the eating disorder examination with children: A pilot study. *International Journal of Eating Disorders, 19*, 391–397.

Bryner, R. W., Toffle, R. C., Ulrich, I. H., & Yeater, R. A. (1997). The effects of exercise intensity on body composition, weight loss, and dietary composition in women. *Journal of American College of Nutrition, 16*, 68–73.

Buchwald, H., Avidor, Y., Braunwald, E., Jensen, M. D., Pories, W., Fahrbach, K., et al. (2004). Bariatric surgery: A systematic review and meta-analysis. *Journal of the American Medical Association, 292*, 1724–1737.

Buchwald, H., & Buchwald, J. N. (2002). Evolution of operative procedures for the management of morbid obesity: 1950–2000. *Obesity Surgery, 12*, 705–717.

Buchwald, H., & Williams, S. E. (2004). Bariatric surgery worldwide 2003. *Obesity Surgery, 14*, 1157–1164.

Buhl, K. M., Gallagher, D., Hoy, K., Matthews, D. E., & Heymsfield, S. B. (1995). Unexplained disturbance in body weight regulation: Diagnostic outcome assessed by doubly labeled water and body composition analyses in obese patients reporting low energy intakes. *Journal of the American Dietetic Association, 95*, 1393–1400.

Bulik, C. M., Bacanu, S. A., Klump, K. L., et al. (2005). Selection of eating-disorder phenotypes for linkage analysis. *American Journal Medical Genetics B. Neuropsychiatric Genetics, 139*, 81–87.

Bulik, C. M., Devlin, B., Bacanu, S. A., et al. (2003). Significant linkage on chromosome 10p in families with bulimia nervosa. *American Journal of Human Genetics, 72*, 200–207.

Bulik, C. M., Sullivan P. F., Fear, J. L., & Joyce, P. R. (1997a). Eating disorders and antecedent anxiety disorders: A controlled study. *Acta Psychiatrica Scandinavicia, 96*, 101–107.

Bulik C., Sullivan, P. F., Fear, J., & Pickering, A. (1997b). Predictors of the development of bulimia nervosa in women with anorexia nervosa. *Journal of Nervous and Mental Disease, 185*, 704–707.

Bulik, C. M., Sullivan, P. F., & Kendler, K. S. (2000a). An empirical study of the classification of eating disorders. *American Journal of Psychiatry, 157*, 886–895.

Bulik, C. M., Sullivan, P. F., & Kendler, K. S. (2002). Medical and psychiatric morbidity in obese women with and without binge eating. *International Journal of Eating Disorders, 32*, 72–78.

Bulik, C. M., Sullivan, P. F., McKee, M., Weltzin, T. E., & Kaye, W. H. (1994). Characteristics of bulimic women with and without alcohol abuse. *American Journal of Drug and Alcohol Abuse, 20,* 273–283.

Bulik, C. M., Sullivan, P. F., Wade, T. D., et al. (2000b). Twin studies of eating disorders: A review. *International Journal of Eating Disorders, 27,* 1–20.

Bulik, C. M., & Tozzi, F. (2004). Contemporary thinking about the roles of genes and environment in eating disorders. *Epidemiologia e Psichiatria Sociale, 13,* 91–98.

Cachelin, F. M., & Maher, B. A. (1998). Is amenorrhea a critical criterion for anorexia nervosa? *Journal of Psychosomatic Research, 44,* 435–440.

Cachelin, F. M., Striegel-Moore, R. H., Elder, K. A., Pike, K. M., Wilfley, D. E., & Fairburn, C. G. (1999). Natural course of a community sample of women with binge eating disorder. *International Journal of Eating Disorders, 25,* 45–54.

Calle, E. E., Thun, M. J., Petrelli, J. M., Rodriguez, C., & Heath, C.W Jr. (1999). Body-mass index and mortality in a prospective cohort of US adults. *New England Journal of Medicine, 341,* 1097–1105.

Carney, T., Tait, D., Saunders, D., Touyz, S., & Beumont, P. (2003). Institutional options in management of coercion in anorexia treatment: The antipodean experiment. *International Journal of Law and Psychiatry, 26,* 647–675.

Carter, J. C., Aime, A. A., & Mills, J. S. (2001). Assessment of bulimia nervosa: A comparison of interview and self-report questionnaire methods. *International Journal of Eating Disorder, 30,* 187–192.

Carter, J. C., & Fairburn, C. G. (1998). Cognitive-behavioral self-help for binge eating disorder: A controlled effectiveness study. *Journal of Consulting and Clinical Psychology, 66,* 616–623.

Carter, J. C., Olmstead, M. P., Kaplan, A. S., McCabe, R. E., Mills, J. S., & Aime, A. (2003). Self-help for bulimia nervosa: A randomized controlled trial. *American Journal of Psychiatry, 160,* 973–978.

Casey, V. A., Dwyer, J. T., Coleman, K. A., & Valadian, I. (1992). Body mass index from childhood to middle age: A 50-year follow-up. *American Journal of Clinical Nutrition, 56,* 14–18.

Cash, T. F., Morrow, J. A., Hrabosky, J. I., & Perry, A. A. (2004). How has body image changed? A cross-sectional investigation of college women and men from 1983–2001. *Journal of Consulting and Clinical Psychology, 72,* 1081–1089.

Cash, T. F., Winstead, B. A., & Janda, L. H. (1986). The great American shape-up: Body image survey report. *Psychology Today,* April, 30–37.

Casper, R. C., & Davis, J. (1977). On the course of anorexia nervosa. *American Journal of Psychiatry, 134,* 974–978.

Casper, R. C., Eckert, E. D., Halmi, K. A., Goldberg, S. C., & Davis, J. M. (1980). Bulimia: Its incidence and clinical importance in patients with anorexia nervosa. *Archives of General Psychiatry, 37,* 1030–1035.

Castro, J., Gila, A., Puig, J., Rodriguez, S., & Toro, J. (2004). Predictors of rehospitalization after total weight recovery in adolescents with anorexia nervosa. *International Journal of Eating Disorders, 36,* 22–30.

Celio, A. A., Wilfley, D. E., Crow, S. J., Mitchell, J., & Walsh, B. T. (2004). A comparison of the Binge Eating Scale, Questionnaire for Eating and Weight Patterns-Revised, and Eating Disorder Examination Questionnaire with Instructions with the Eating Disorder Examination in the assessment of binge eating disorder and its symptoms. *International Journal of Eating Disorders, 36,* 434–444.

Centre for Pharmaceutical Administration, Health Sciences Authority (2003, May). Drug alerts updates report on sibutramine. (www.hsa.gov.sg/hsa/

CPA/CPA_pharma_drugalerts.
htm#12).

Chambliss, H. O., Finley, C. E., & Blair,
S. N. (2004). Attitudes toward obese
individuals among exercise science
students. *Medicine and Science in Sports
and Exercise, 36,* 468–474.

Chan, J. M., Rimm, E. B., Colditz, G. A.,
Stampfer, M. J., & Willett, W. C. (1994).
Obesity, fat distribution, and weight
gain as risk factors for clinical diabetes
in men. *Diabetes Care, 17,* 961–969.

Christou, N. V., Sampalis, J. S., Liberman,
M., Look, D., Auger, W. S., McLean,
A. P., et al. (2004). Surgery decreases
long-term mortality, morbidity, and
health care use in morbidly obese
patients. *Annals of Surgery, 240,*
416–423.

Clapham, J. C., Arch, J. R., & Tadayyon, M.
(2001). Anti-obesity drugs: A critical
review of current therapies and future
opportunities. *Pharmacology and
Therapeutics, 89,* 81–121.

Colditz, G. A. (1992). Economic costs of
obesity. *American Journal of Clinical
Nutrition, 55,* 503S–507S.

Colditz, G. A., Willett, W. C., Rotnitzky,
A., & Manson, J. E. (1995). Weight gain
as a risk factor for clinical diabetes
mellitus in women. *Annals of Internal
Medicine, 122,* 481–486.

Cole, T. J., Bellizzi, M. C., Flegal, K. M., &
Dietz, W. H. (2000). Establishing a
standard definition for child
overweight and obesity worldwide:
International Survey. *British Medical
Journal, 320,* 1240–1243.

Collier, D. A., & Treasure, J. L. (2004). The
aetiology of eating disorders. *British
Journal of Psychiatry, 185,* 363–365.

Cooper, P. J., Coker, S., & Fleming, C.
(1996). An evaluation of the efficacy of
supervised cognitive behavioral self-
help bulimia nervosa. *Journal of
Psychosomatic Research, 40,* 281–287.

Cooper, P. J., & Fairburn, C. G. (1993).
Confusion over the core

psychopathology of bulimia nervosa.
*International Journal of Eating Disorders,
13,* 385–389.

Cooper, P. J., Watkins, B., Bryant-Waugh,
R., & Lask, B. (2002). The nosological
status of early onset anorexia nervosa.
Psychological Medicine, 32, 873–880.

Cottam, D. R., Nguyen, N. T., Eid, G. M., &
Schauer, P. R. (2005). The impact of
laparoscopy on bariatric surgery,
Surgical Endoscopy 19, 621–627.

Crago, M., Shisslak, C. M., & Estes, L. S.
(1996). Eating disturbances among
American minority groups: A review.
*International Journal of Eating Disorders,
19,* 239–248.

Craighead, L. (1984). Sequencing of
behavior therapy and pharmacotherapy
for obesity. *Journal of Consulting and
Clinical Psychology, 52,* 190–199.

Craighead, L. W., & Agras, W. S. (1991).
Mechanisms of action in cognitive-
behavioral and pharmacological
interventions for obesity and bulimia
nervosa. *Journal of Consulting and
Clinical Psychology, 59,* 115–125.

Craighead, L. W., Stunkard, A. J., &
O'Brien, R. (1981). Behavioral therapy
and pharmacotherapy of obesity.
Archives of General Psychiatry, 38,
763–768.

Cramer, P., & Steinwert, T. (1998). Thin is
good, fat is bad: How early does it
begin? *Journal of Applied Developmental
Psychology, 19,* 429–451.

Crisp, A. H., Callender, J. S., Halek, C., &
Hsu, L. K. G. (1992). Long-term
mortality in anorexia nervosa: A 20-
year follow-up of the St. George's and
Aberdeen cohorts. *British Journal of
Psychiatry, 161,* 104–107.

Crow, S. J., Keel, P. K., & Kendall, D.
(1998). Eating disorders and insulin-
dependent diabetes mellitus.
Psychosomatics, 39, 233–243.

Crow, S., Kendall, D., Praus, B., & Thuras,
P. (2001). Binge eating and other
psychopathology in patients with type

II diabetes mellitus. *International Journal of Eating Disorders, 30,* 222–226.

Crow, S., Mussel, M. P., Peterson, C., Knopke, A., & Mitchell, J. (1999). Prior treatment received by patients with bulimia nervosa. *International Journal of Eating Disorders, 25,* 39–44.

Crow, S. J., Peterson, C. B., Levine, A. S., Thuras, P., & Mitchell, J. E. (2004). A survey of binge eating and obesity treatment practices among primary care providers. *International Journal of Eating Disorders, 35,* 348–353.

Dansky, B. S., Brewerton, T. D., Kilpatrick, D. G., O'Neil, P. M., Resnick, H. S., Best, C. L., et al. (1998). The nature and prevalence of binge eating disorder in a national sample of women. In T. A. Widiger, A. J. Frances, H. A. Pincus, R. Ross, M. B. First, W. Davis, & M. Kline (Eds.), *DSM-IV sourcebook* (pp. 515–532). Washington, DC: American Psychological Association Press.

Dare, C., & Eisler, I. (1997). Family therapy for anorexia nervosa. In D. M. Garner & P. E. Garfinkel (Eds.), *Handbook of treatment for eating disorders* (2nd ed., pp. 307–324). New York: Guilford Press.

Dare, C., Eisler, I., Russell, G., Treasure, J., & Dodge, L. (2001). Psychological therapies for adults with anorexia nervosa: Randomised controlled trial of out-patient treatments. *British Journal of Psychiatry, 178,* 216–221.

Davidson, M. H., Hauptman, J., Digirolamo, M., Foreyt, J. P., Halsted, C. H., Heber, D., et al. (1999). Weight control and risk factor reduction in obese subjects treated for 2 years with orlistat: A randomized controlled trial. *Journal of the American Medical Association, 281,* 235–242.

Davis, C., Katzman, D. K., Kaptein, S., Kirsh, C., Brewer, H., Kalmbach, K., et al. (1997). The prevalence of high-level exercise in the eating disorders:

Etiological implications. *Comprehensive Psychiatry, 38,* 321–326.

Davis, C., Kennedy, S. H., Ralevski, E., Dionne, M., Brewer, H., Neitzert, C., et al. (1995). Obsessive compulsiveness and physical activity in anorexia nervosa and high-level exercising. *Journal of Psychosomatic Research, 39,* 967–976.

Deitel, M., & Shikora, S. A. (2002). The development of surgical treatment of morbid obesity. *Journal of the American College of Nutrition, 21,* 365–371.

DeLany, J. P., Bray, G. A., Harsha, D. W., & Volaufova, J. (2002). Energy expenditure in preadolescent African American and white boys and girls: The Baton Rouge Children's Study. *American Journal of Clinical Nutrition, 75,* 705–713.

Derosa, G., Cicero, A. F., Murdolo, G., Ciccarelli, L., & Fogari, R. (2004). Comparison of metabolic effects of orlistat and sibutramine in Type 2 diabetic obese patients. *Diabetes, Nutrition, and Metabolism, 17,* 222–229.

Derosa, G., Cicero, A. F., Murdolo, G., Piccinni, M. N., Fogari, E., Bertone, G., et al. (2005). Efficacy and safety comparative evaluation of orlistat and sibutramine treatment in hypertensive obese patients. *Diabetes, Obesity, and Metabolism, 7,* 47–55.

Despres, J. P. (2002). The metabolic syndrome. In C. G. Fairburn & K. D. Brownell (Eds.), *Eating disorders and obesity: A comprehensive handbook* (2nd ed., pp. 477–483). New York: Guilford Press.

Despres, J. P., Moorjani, S., Lupien, P. J., Tremblay, A., Nadeau, A., & Bouchard, C. (1990). Regional distribution of body fat, plasma lipoproteins, and cardiovascular disease. *Arteriosclerosis, 10,* 497–511.

Devlin, B., Bacanu, S. A., Klump, K. A., Bulik, C. M., Fichter, M. M., Halmi, K. A., et al. (2002). Linkage analysis of anorexia nervosa incorporating behavioral covariates. *Human Molecular Genetics, 15,* 689–696.

Devlin, M. J., Goldfein, J. A., Petkova, E., Jiang, H., Raizman, P. S., Wolk, S., et al. (2005). Cognitive behavioral therapy and fluoxetine as adjuncts to group behavioral therapy for binge eating disorders. *Obesity Research, 13,* 1077–1088.

de Zwaan, M., Burgard, M. A., Schenck, C. H., & Mitchell, J. E. (2003). Night time eating: A review of the literature. *European Eating Disorders Review, 11,* 7–24.

de Zwann, M., Nutzinger, D. O., & Schoenbeck, G. (1992). Binge eating in overweight women. *Comprehensive Psychiatry, 33,* 256–261.

Diabetes Prevention Research Group (DPRG, 2002). Reduction in the evidence of type 2 diabetes with lifestyle intervention or metformin. *New England Journal of Medicine, 346,* 393–403.

Diliberti, N., Bordi, P. L., Conklin, M. T., Roe, L. S., & Rolls, B. J. (2004). Increased portion size leads to increased energy intake in a restaurant meal. *Obesity Research, 12,* 562–568.

DiPietro, L., Mossberg, H. O., & Stunkard, A. J. (1994). A 40-year history of overweight children in Stockholm: Lifetime overweight, morbidity, and mortality. *International Journal of Obesity, 18,* 585–590.

Drent, M. L., & Van der Veen, E. A. (1993). Lipase inhibition: A novel concept in the treatment of obesity. *International Journal of Obesity, 17,* 241–244.

Drury, C. A., & Louis, M. (2002). Exploring the association between body weight, stigma of obesity, and health care avoidance. *Journal of the American Academy of Nurse Practitioners, 14,* 554–561.

Duncan, J. J., Gordon, N. F., & Scott, C. B. (1991). Women walking for health and fitness: How much is enough? *Journal of the American Medical Association, 266,* 3295–3299.

Dunn, A. L., Marcus, S. H., Kampert, J. B., Garcia, M. E., Kohl, H. W., & Blair, S. N. (1999). Comparison of lifestyle and structured interventions to increase physical activity and cardiorespiratory fitness: A randomized trial. *Journal of American Medical Association, 281,* 327–334.

Durand, M. A., & King, M. (2003). Specialist treatment versus self-help for bulimia nervosa: A randomised controlled trial in general practice. *British Journal of General Practice, 53,* 371–377.

Eating Disorders Commission (2005). Part IV: Eating disorders. In D. L. Evans, E. Foa, R. Gur, H. Hendin, C. P. O'Brien, M. E. P. Seligman, et al. (Eds.), *Treating and preventing adolescent mental health disorders: What we know and what we don't know.* Oxford: Oxford University Press.

Eckel, R. H., & Krauss, R. H. (1998). American Heart Association call to action: Obesity as a major risk factor for coronary heart disease. AHA Nutrition Committee. *Circulation, 97,* 2099–2100.

Eckert, E. D., Halmi, K. A., Marchi, P., Grove, W., & Crosby, R. (1995). Ten-year follow-up of anorexia nervosa: Clinical course and outcome. *Psychological Medicine, 25,* 143–156.

Eddy, K. T., Keel, P. K., Dorer, D. J., Delinsky, S. S., Franko, D. L., & Herzog, D. B. (2002). Longitudinal comparison of anorexia nervosa subtypes. *International Journal of Eating Disorders, 31,* 191–201.

Eisler, I., Dare, C., Hodes, M., Russell, G., Dodge, E., & Le Grange, D. (2000). Family therapy for adolescent anorexia nervosa: The results of a controlled comparison of two family interventions. *Journal of Child Psychology and Psychiatry, 41,* 727–736.

Eisler, I., Dare, C. Russell, G., Szmukler, G., le Grange, D., & Dodge, E. (1997). Family and individual therapy in anorexia nervosa: A 5-year follow-up. *Archives of General Psychiatry, 54,* 1025–1030.

Elder, K. A., Grilo, C. M., Masheb, R. M., Rothschild, B. S., Burke-Martindale, C. H., & Brody, M. L. (2006). A comparison of two self-report instruments for assessing binge eating in bariatric surgery candidates. *Behaviour Research and Therapy, 44,* 545–560.

Epstein, L. H., Myers, M. D., Raynor, H. A., & Saelens, B. E. (1998). Treatment of pediatric obesity. *Pediatrics, 101,* 554–570.

Epstein, L. H., Valoski, A. M., Vara, L. S., McCurley, J., Wisniewski, L., Kalarchian, M. A., et al. (1995). Effects of decreasing sedentary behavior and increasing activity on weight change in obese children. *Health Psychology, 14,* 109–115.

Epstein, L. H., Valoski, A. M., Wing, R. R., & McCurley, J. (1994). Ten year outcomes of behavioral family-based treatment for childhood obesity. *Health Psychology, 13,* 373–383.

Epstein, L. H., Wing, R. R., Koeske, R., & Valoski, A. (1984). The effects of diet plus exercise on weight change in parents and children. *Journal of Consulting and Clinical Psychology, 52,* 427–429.

Epstein, L. H., Wing, R. R., Koeske, R., & Valoski, A. (1985). A comparison of lifestyle exercise, aerobic exercise and calisthenics on weight loss in obese children. *Behavior Therapy, 16,* 345–356.

Expert Committee on the Diagnosis and Classification of Diabetes Mellitus (2003). Follow-up report on the diagnosis of diabetes mellitus. *Diabetes Care, 26,* 3160–3167.

Fairburn, C. G. (1997). Interpersonal psychotherapy for bulimia nervosa. In D. M. Garner & P. E. Garfinkel (Eds.), *Handbook of treatment for eating disorders* (pp. 278–294). New York: Guilford Press.

Fairburn, C. G., Agras, W. S., Walsh, B. T., Wilson, G. T., & Stice, E. (2004a). Early change in treatment predicts outcome in bulimia nervosa. *American Journal of Psychiatry, 161,* 2322–2324.

Fairburn, C. G., Agras, W. S., Walsh, B. T., Wilson, G. T., & Stice, E. (2004b). Prediction of outcome in bulimia nervosa by early change in treatment. *American Journal of Psychiatry, 161,* 2322–2324.

Fairburn, C. G., & Beglin, S. J. (1990). Studies of the epidemiology of bulimia nervosa. *American Journal of Psychiatry, 147,* 401–408.

Fairburn, C. G., & Beglin, S. J. (1994). Assessment of eating disorders: Interview or self-report questionnaire? *International Journal of Eating Disorders, 16,* 363–370.

Fairburn, C. G., & Bohn, K. (in press). Eating disorder NOS (EDNOS): An example of the troublesome "not otherwise specified" (NOS) category in DSM-IV. *Behaviour Research and Therapy.*

Fairburn, C. G., & Cooper, P. J. (1982). Self-induced vomiting and bulimia nervosa: An undetected problem. *British Medical Journal, 284,* 1153–1155.

Fairburn, C. G., & Cooper, P. J. (1984). The clinical features of bulimia nervosa. *British Journal of Psychiatry, 144,* 238–246.

Fairburn, C. G., & Cooper, Z. (1993). The schedule of the Eating Disorder Examination. In C. G. Fairburn & G. T. Wilson (Eds.), *Binge eating: Nature, assessment, and treatment.* New York: Guilford Press.

Fairburn, C. G., Cooper, Z., Doll, H. A., Norman, P., & O'Connor, M. (2000). The natural course of bulimia nervosa and binge eating disorder in young women. *Archives of General Psychiatry,* 57, 659–665.

Fairburn, C. G., Cooper, Z., & Shafran, R. (2003a). Cognitive behaviour therapy for eating disorders: A "transdiagnostic" theory and treatment. *Behaviour Research and Therapy, 41,* 509–529.

Fairburn, C. G., Doll, H. A., Welch, S., Hay, P. J., Davies, B. A., O'Connor, M. E. (1998). Risk factors for binge eating disorder: A community-based, case-control study. *Archives of General Psychiatry, 55,* 425–432.

Fairburn, C. G., & Harrison, P. J. (2003). Eating disorders. *Lancet, 361,* 407–416.

Fairburn, C. G., Jones, R., Peveler, R. C., Carr, S. J., Hope, R. A., & O'Connor, M. E. (1993a). Psychotherapy and bulimia nervosa: Longer-term effects of interpersonal psychotherapy, behavior therapy, and cognitive-behavior therapy. *Archives of General Psychiatry, 50,* 419–428.

Fairburn, C. G., Jones, R., Peveler, R. C., Carr, S. J., Solomon, R. A., O'Connor, M. E., et al. (1991). Three psychological treatments for bulimia nervosa: A comparative trial. *Archives of General Psychiatry, 48,* 463–469.

Fairburn, C. G., Marcus, M. D., & Wilson, G. T. (1993b). Cognitive behavior therapy for binge eating and bulimia nervosa: A comprehensive treatment manual. In C. G. Fairburn & G. T. Wilson (Eds.), *Binge eating: Nature, assessment, and treatment* (pp. 361–404). New York: Guilford Press.

Fairburn, C. G., Stice, E., Cooper, Z., Doll, H. A., Norman, P. A., & O'Connor, M. E. (2003b). Understanding persistence in bulimia nervosa: A 5-year naturalistic study. *Journal of Consulting and Clinical Psychology, 71,* 103–109.

Fairburn, C. G., & Walsh, B. T. (2002). Atypical eating disorders (eating disorder not otherwise specified). In C. G. Fairburn, & K. D. Brownell (Eds.), *Eating disorders and obesity: A comprehensive handbook* (2nd ed., pp. 171–177). New York: Guilford Press.

Fairburn, C. G., Welch, S. L., Doll, H. A., & Davies, B. A. (1997). Risk factors for bulimia nervosa: A community-based case-control study. *Archives of General Psychiatry, 54,* 509–517.

Fairburn, C. G., Welch, S. L, & Hay, P. J. (1993c). The classification of recurrent overeating: The "binge eating disorder" proposal. *International Journal of Eating Disorders, 13,* 155–159.

Fairburn, C. G., Welch, S. L., Norman, P. A., O'Connor, M. E., & Doll, H. A. (1996). Bias and bulimia nervosa: How typical are clinic cases? *American Journal of Psychiatry, 153,* 386–391.

Feingold, A., & Mazzalla, R. (1998). Gender differences in body image are increasing. *Psychological Science, 9,* 190–195.

Ferster, C. B., Nurnberger, J. I., & Levitt, E. E. (1962). The control of eating. *Journal of Mathetics, 1,* 87–109.

Fichter, M. M. (2005). *Six-year course and outcome of binge eating disorder.* Paper presented at the Annual Meeting of the Eating Disorder Research Society, Toronto, Canada.

Fichter M. M., Leibl, K., Rief, W., Brunner, E., Schmidt-Auberger S., & Engel, R. R. (1991). Fluoxetine versus placebo: A double-blind study with bulimic inpatients undergoing intensive psychotherapy. *Pharmacopsychiatry, 24,* 1–7.

Fichter, M. M., & Quadflieg, N. (1997). Six-year course of bulimia nervosa. *International Journal of Eating Disorders, 22,* 361–384.

Fichter, M. M., & Quadflieg, N. (2004). Twelve-year course of bulimia nervosa. *Psychological Medicine, 34,* 1395–1406.

Fichter, M. M., Quadflieg, N., & Brandl, B. (1993). Recurrent overeating: An empirical comparison of binge eating disorder, bulimia nervosa, and obesity.

International Journal of Eating Disorders, 14, 1–16.

Fichter, M. M., Quadflieg, N., & Rehm, J. (2003). Predicting the outcome of eating disorders using structural equation modeling. International Journal of Eating Disorders, 34, 292–313.

First, M. B., Spitzer, R. L., Gibbon, M., & Williams, J. B. W. (1996). Structured clinical interview for DSM-IV Axis I disorders – patient Edition (SCID-I/P, Version 2.0). New York: Biometrics Research Department, New York State Psychiatric Institute.

Fitzgibbon, M. L., & Blackman, L. R. (2000). Binge eating disorder and bulimia nervosa: Differences in the quality and quantity of binge eating episodes. International Journal of Eating Disorders, 27, 238–243.

Flegal, K. M., Graubard, B. I., Williamson, D. F., & Gail, M. H. (2005). Excess deaths associated with underweight, overweight, and obesity. Journal of the American Medical Association, 293, 1861–1867.

Fluoxetine Bulimia Nervosa Collaborative Study Group (FBNCSG; 1992). Fluoxetine in the treatment of bulimia nervosa. A multicenter, placebo-controlled, double-blind trial. Archives of General Psychiatry, 49, 139–147.

Folsom, A. R., Kushi, L. H., Anderson, K. E., Mink, P. J., Olson, J. E., Hong, C. P., et al. (2000). Associations of general and abdominal obesity with multiple health outcomes in older women. Archives of Internal Medicine, 160, 2117–2128.

Fontaine, K. R., Faith, M. S., Allison, D. B., & Cheskin, L. J. (1998). Body weight and health care among women in the general population. Archives of Family Medicine, 7, 381–384.

Fontaine, K. R., Redden, D. T., Wang, C., Westfall, A. O., & Allison, D. B. (2003). Years of life lost due to obesity. Journal of the American Medical Association, 289, 187–193.

Ford, E. S., Giles, W. H., & Dietz, W. H. (2002). Prevalence of the metabolic syndrome among US adults: Findings from the third National Health and Nutrition Examination Survey. Journal of the American Medical Association, 287, 356–359.

Foster, G. A., Wadden, T. A., & Vogt, R. A. (1997a). Body image in obese women before, during, and after weight loss treatment. Health Psychology, 16, 226–229.

Foster, G. A., Wadden, T. A., Vogt, R. A., & Brewer, G. (1997b). What is a reasonable weight loss? Patients' expectations and evaluations of obesity treatment outcomes. Journal of Consulting and Clinical Psychology, 65, 79–85.

Foster, G. D., Wyatt, H. R., Hill, J. O., McGuckin, B. G., Brill, C., Mohammed, B. S., et al. (2003). A randomized trial of a low-carbohydrate diet for obesity. New England Journal of Medicine, 348, 2082–2090.

Fox, C., Esparza, J., Nicolson, M., Bennett, P. H., Shulz, L. O., Valencia, M. E., et al. (1999). Plasma leptin concentrations in Pima Indians living in drastically different environments. Diabetes Care, 22, 413–417.

Franko, D. L., Blais, M. A., Becker, A. E., Delinsky, S. S., Greenwood, D. N., Flores, A. T., et al. (2001). Pregnancy complications and neonatal outcomes in women with eating disorders. American Journal of Psychiatry, 158, 1461–1466.

Franko, D. L., & Spurrell, E. B. (2000). Detection and management of eating disorders during pregnancy. Obstetrics and Gynecology, 95, 942–946.

Friedman, M. A., & Brownell, K. D. (1995). Psychological correlates of obesity: Moving to the next research generation. Psychological Bulletin, 117, 3–17.

Garfinkel, P. E., Kennedy, S., & Kaplan, A. (1995). Views on classification and diagnosis of eating disorders. *Canadian Journal of Psychiatry, 40,* 445–456.

Garfinkel, P. E., Lin, E., Goering, P., Spegg, C., Goldbloom, D. S., Kennedy, S., et al. (1995). Bulimia nervosa in a Canadian community sample: Prevalence and comparison of subgroups. *American Journal of Psychiatry, 152,* 1052–1058.

Garfinkel, P. E., Lin, E., Goering, P., Spegg, C., Goldbloom, D., Kennedy, S., et al. (1996). Should amenorrhea be a necessary for the diagnosis of anorexia nervosa? *British Journal of Psychiatry, 168,* 500–506.

Garfinkel, P. E., Moldofsky, H., & Garner, D. M. (1980). The heterogeneity of anorexia nervosa. Bulimia as a distinct subgroup. *Archives of General Psychiatry, 37,* 1036–1040.

Garn, S. M., Sullivan, T. V., & Hawthorne, V. M. (1989). Fatness and obesity of the parents of obese individuals. *American Journal of Clinical Nutrition, 50,* 1308–1313.

Garner, D. M. (1997). The 1997 body image survey results. *Psychology Today,* January/February, 30–44, 75–80, 84.

Garner, D. M., Rockert, W., Davis, R., Garner, M. V., Olmsted, M. P., & Eagle, M. (1993). Comparison of cognitive-behavioral and supportive-expressive therapy for bulimia nervosa. *American Journal of Psychiatry, 150,* 37–46.

Geier, A. B., Schwartz, M. B., & Brownell, K. D. (2003). "Before and after" diet advertisements escalate weight stigma. *Eating and Weight Disorders, 8,* 282–288.

Geist, R., Heinmaa, M., Stephens, D., Davis, R., Katzman, D. K. (2000). Comparison of family therapy and family group psychoeducation in adolescents with anorexia nervosa. *Canadian Journal of Psychiatry, 45,* 173–178.

Gladis, M. M., Wadden, T. A., Foster, G. D., Vogt, R. A., & Wingate, B. J. (1998a). A comparison of two approaches to the assessment of binge eating in obesity. *International Journal of Eating Disorders, 23,* 17–26.

Gladis, M. M., Wadden, T. A., Vogt, R., Foster, G., Kuehnel, R. H., & Bartlett, S. J. (1998b). Behavioral treatment of obese binge eaters: Do they need different care? *Journal of Psychosomatic Research, 44,* 375–384.

Glasgow, R. E., Klesges, L. M., Dzewaltowski, D., Bull, S. S., Estabrooks, P. (2004). The future of health behavior change research: What is needed to improve translation of research into health promoting practice? *Annals of Behavioral Medicine, 27,* 3–12.

Glasgow, R. E., Lichtenstein, E., & Marcus, A. (2003). Why don't we see more translation of health promotion research to practice? Rethinking the efficacy to effectiveness transition. *American Journal of Public Health, 93,* 1261–1267.

Gokcel, A., Gumurdulu, Y., Karakose, H., Melek Ertorer, E., Tanaci, N., BascilTutuncu, N., et al. (2002). Evaluation of the safety and efficacy of sibutramine, orlistat, and metformin in the treatment of obesity. *Diabetes, Obesity, and Metabolism, 4,* 49–55.

Goldbloom, D. S., Olmstead, M., Davis, R., Clewes, J., Heinmaa, M., Rockert, W., et al. (1997). A randomized controlled trial of fluoxetine and cognitive-behavioral therapy for bulimia nervosa: Short-term outcome. *Behaviour Research and Therapy, 35,* 803–811.

Goldfein, J. A., Devlin, M. J., & Spitzer, R. L. (2000). Cognitive behavioral therapy for the treatment of binge eating disorder: What constitutes success? *American Journal of Psychiatry, 157,* 1051–1056.

Goldfield, A., & Chrisler, J. C. (1995). Body stereotyping and stigmatization of obese persons by first graders. *Perceptual and Motor Skills, 81,* 909–910.

Goldstein, D. J. (1992). Beneficial health effects of modest weight loss. *International Journal of Obesity and Related Metabolic Disorders, 16,* 397–415.

Goldstein, D. J., Wilson, M. G., Thompson, V. L., Potvin, J. H., & Rampey, A. H. (1995). Long-term fluoxetine treatment of bulimia. The Fluoxetine Bulimia Nervosa Research Group. *British Journal of Psychiatry, 166,* 660–666.

Goodman, E., & Whitaker, R. C. (2002). A prospective study of the role of depression in the development and persistence of adolescent obesity. *Pediatrics, 109,* 497–504.

Goodrick, G. K., Poston II, W. S., Kimball, K. T., Reeves, R. S., & Foreyt, J. P. (1998). Nondieting versus dieting treatment for overweight binge-eating women. *Journal of Consulting and Clinical Psychology, 66,* 363–368.

Gortmaker, S. L., Must, A., Perrin, J. M., Sobol, A. M., & Dietz, W. H. (1993). Social and economic consequences of overweight in adolescence and young adulthood. *New England Journal of Medicine, 329,* 1008–1012.

Gowers, S. G., Weetman, J., Shore, A., Hossain, F., & Elvins, R. (2000). Impact of hospitalization on the outcome of adolescent anorexia nervosa. *British Journal of Psychiatry, 176,* 138–141.

Greenberg, B. S., Eastin, M., Hofschire, L., Lachlan, K., & Brownell, K. D. (2003). Portrayals of overweight and obese individuals on commercial television. *American Journal of Public Health, 93,* 1342–1348.

Greenfeld, D., Mickley, D., Quinlan, D., & Roloff, P. (1995). Hypokalemia in outpatients with eating disorders. *American Journal of Psychiatry, 152,* 60–63.

Greenstein, R. J., & Rabner, J. G. (1995). Is adolescent gastric-restrictive antiobesity surgery warranted? *Obesity Surgery, 5,* 138–144.

Grice, D. E., Halmi, K. A., Fichter, M. M., et al. (2002). Evidence for a susceptibility gene for anorexia nervosa on chromosome 1. *American Journal of Human Genetics, 70,* 787–792.

Griffin, W. O., Young, V. L., & Stevenson, C. C. (1977). A prospective comparison of gastric and jejuno-ileal procedures for morbid obesity. *Annals of Surgery, 186,* 500–509.

Grilo, C. M. (1994). Physical activity and obesity. *Biomedicine and Pharmacotherapy, 48,* 127–136.

Grilo, C. M. (1998). The assessment and treatment of binge eating disorder. *Practice of Psychiatry and Behavioral Health, 4,* 191–201.

Grilo, C. M. (2000). Self-help and guided self-help treatments for BN and BED. *Journal of Psychiatric Practice, 6,* 18–26.

Grilo, C. M. (2002). Binge eating disorder. In C. G. Fairburn & K. D. Brownell (Eds.), *Comprehensive textbook of obesity and eating disorders* (2nd ed., pp. 178–182). New York: Guilford Press.

Grilo, C. M. (2004). Pharmacotherapy for binge eating disorder. Plenary presentation at the Annual Meeting of the North American Association for the Study of Obesity (NAASO), Las Vegas, Nevada.

Grilo, C. M. (2005). Structured instruments. In J. E. Mitchell, & C. Peterson (Eds.), *The assessment of patients with eating disorders.* New York: Guilford Press.

Grilo, C. M., Becker, D. F., Levy, K. N., Walker, M. L, Edell, W. S., & McGlashan, T. H. (1995a). Eating disorders with and without substance use disorders: A comparative study of inpatients. *Comprehensive Psychiatry, 36,* 312–317.

Grilo, C. M., & Brownell, K. D. (1998). Interventions for weight management. In *ACSM resource manual for guidelines for exercise testing and prescription* (3rd ed.). Philadelphia: Lea & Febiger.

Grilo, C. M., & Brownell, K. D. (2001). Interventions for weight management. In: *ACSM resource manual for guidelines for exercise testing and prescription* (4th ed.). Philadelphia: Lea & Fibiger.

Grilo, C. M., Brownell, K. D., & Stunkard, A. J. (1993). The metabolic and psychological importance of exercise in weight control. In A. J. Stunkard & T. A. Wadden (Eds.), *Obesity: Theory and therapy* (pp. 253–273). New York: Raven Press.

Grilo, C. M., Devlin, M. J., Cachelin, F. M., & Yanovski, S. (1997). Report of the National Institutes of Health Workshop on the Development of Research Priorities in Eating Disorders. *Psychopharmacology Bulletin, 33,* 321–333.

Grilo, C. M., Levy, K. N., Becker, D. F., Edell, W. S., & McGlashan, T. H. (1995b). Eating disorders in female inpatients with versus without substance use disorders. *Addictive Behaviors, 20,* 255–260.

Grilo, C. M., Levy, K. N., Becker, D. F., Edell, W. S., & McGlashan, T. H. (1996). Comorbidity of DSM-III-R axis I and axis II diagnoses among female inpatients with eating disorders. *Psychiatric Services, 47,* 426–429.

Grilo, C. M., Lozano, C., & Elder, K. A. (2005). Inter-rates and test-retest reliability of the Spanish language version of the Eating Disorder Examination Interview: Clinical and research implications. *Journal of Psychiatric Practice 11,* 231–240.

Grilo, C. M., Lozano, C., & Masheb, R. M. (2005). Ethnicity and sampling bias in binge eating disorder. *International Journal of Eating Disorders, 38,* 257–262.

Grilo, C. M., & Masheb, R. M. (2000). Onset of dieting vs binge eating in outpatients with binge eating disorder. *International Journal of Obesity, 24,* 404–409.

Grilo, C. M., & Masheb, R. M. (2004). Night-time eating in men and women with binge eating disorder. *Behaviour Research and Therapy, 42,* 397–407.

Grilo, C. M., & Masheb, R. M. (2005). A randomized controlled comparison of guided self-help cognitive behavioral therapy and behavioral weight loss for binge eating disorder. *Behaviour Research and Therapy, 43,* 1509–1525.

Grilo, C. M., Masheb, R. M., & Berman, R. M. (2001). Subtyping women with bulimia nervosa along dietary and negative affect dimensions: a replication in a treatment-seeking sample. *Eating and Weight Disorders, 6,* 53–58.

Grilo, C. M., Masheb, R. M., Brody, M., Toth, C., Burke-Martindale, C. H., & Rothschild, B. S. (2005a). Childhood maltreatment in extremely obese male and female bariatric surgery candidates. *Obesity Research, 13,* 123–130.

Grilo, C. M., Masheb, R., Lozano-Blanco, C., & Barry, T. (2004a). Reliability of the Eating Disorder Examination in patients with binge eating disorder. *International Journal of Eating Disorders, 35,* 80–85.

Grilo, C. M., Masheb, R. M., & Salant, S. L. (2005b). Cognitive behavioral therapy guided self-help and orlistat for the treatment of binge eating disorder: A randomized double-blind placebo-controlled trial. *Biological Psychiatry, 57,* 1193–1201.

Grilo, C. M., Masheb, R. M., & Wilson, G. T. (2001a). Subtyping binge eating disorder. *Journal of Consulting and Clinical Psychology, 69,* 1066–1072.

Grilo, C. M., Masheb, R. M., & Wilson, G. T. (2001b). A comparison of different methods for assessing the features of eating disorders in patients with binge eating disorder. *Journal of Consulting and Clinical Psychology, 69,* 317–322.

Grilo, C. M., Masheb, R. M., & Wilson, G. T.

(2001c). Different methods for assessing the features of eating disorders in patients with binge eating disorder: A replication. *Obesity Research, 9,* 418–422.

Grilo, C. M., Masheb, R. M., & Wilson, G. T. (2005c). Efficacy of cognitive-behavioral therapy and fluoxetine for the treatment of binge eating disorder: A randomized double-blind placebo-controlled comparison. *Biological Psychiatry, 57,* 301–309.

Grilo, C. M., & Pogue-Geile, M. F. (1991). The nature of environmental influences on weight and obesity: A behavior genetic analysis. *Psychological Bulletin, 110,* 520–537.

Grilo, C. M., Sanislow, C. A., Shea, M. T., Skodol, A. E., Stout, R. L., Pagano, M. E., et al. (2003a). The natural course of bulimia nervosa and eating disorder not otherwise classified is not influenced by personality disorders. *International Journal of Eating Disorders, 34,* 319–330.

Grilo, C. M., Sanislow, C. A., Skodol, A. E., Gunderson, J. G., Stout, R. L., Shea, M. T., et al. (2003b). Do eating disorders co-occur with personality disorders? Comparison groups matter. *International Journal of Eating Disorders, 33,* 155–164.

Grilo, C. M., & Shiffman, S. (1994). Longitudinal investigation of the abstinence violation effect in binge eaters. *Journal of Consulting and Clinical Psychology, 62,* 611–619.

Grilo, C. M., White, M. A., Masheb, R. M., Rothschild, B. S., & Burke-Martindale, C. H. (2006). Relation of childhood sexual abuse and other forms of maltreatment to 12-month postoperative outcomes in extremely obese gastric bypass patients. *Obesity Surgery, 16,* 454–460.

Grinspoon, S., Thomas, L., Miller, K., Herzog, D., & Klibanski, A. (2002). Effects of recombinant human IGF-I and oral contraceptive administration on bone density in anorexia nervosa. *Journal of Clinical Endocrinology, 87,* 2883–2891.

Grinspoon, S., Thomas, E., Pitts, S., Gross, E., Mickley, D., Miller, K., et al. (2000). Prevalence and predictive factors for regional osteopenia in women with anorexia nervosa. *Annals of Internal Medicine, 133,* 790–794.

Grunbaum, J. A., Kann, L., Kinchen, S., Ross, J. G., Hawkins, J., Lowry, R., et al. (2004). Youth risk behavior surveillance – United States, 2003. *Morbidity and Mortality Weekly Report, 53,* 1–96.

Grunbaum, J., Kann, L., Kinchen, S. A., Williams, B., Ross, J. G., Lowry, R., et al. (2002). Youth risk behavior surveillance – United States, 2001. *Journal of School Health, 72,* 313–328.

Grundy, S. M., Brewer, H. B., Cleeman, J. I., Smith, S. C., & Lenfant, D. (2004). Definition of metabolic syndrome: Report of the National, Heart, Lung, and Blood Institute/American Heart Association conference on scientific issues related to definition. *Circulation, 109,* 433–438.

Guo, S. S., Wu, W., Chumlea, W. C., & Roche, A. F. (2002). Predicting overweight and obesity in adulthood from body mass index values in childhood and adolescence. *American Journal of Clinical Nutrition, 76,* 653–658.

Guss, J. L, Kissileff, H. R., Devlin, M. J., Zimmerli, E., & Walsh, B. T. (2002). Binge size increases with body mass index in women with binge-eating disorder. *Obesity Research, 10,* 1021–1029.

Hager, J., Dina, C., Francke, S., Dubois, S., Houari, M., Vatin, V., et al. (1998). A genome-wide scan for human obesity genes reveals a major susceptibility locus on chromosome 10. *Nature Genetics, 20,* 304–308.

Hall, R. C., Blakey, R. E., & Hall, A. K. (1992). Bulimia nervosa. Four

uncommon subtypes. *Psychosomatics,*
33, 428–436.

Halmi, K. A., Agras, W. S., Crow, S.,
Mitchell, J., Wilson, J. E., Bryson, S. W.,
et al. (2005). Predictors of treatment
acceptance and completion in anorexia
nervosa: Implications for future study
designs. *Archives of General Psychiatry,*
62, 776–781.

Halmi, K. A., Casper, R. C., Eckert, E. D.,
Goldberg, S. C., & Davis, J. M. (1979).
Unique features associated with age of
onset of anorexia nervosa. *Psychiatry*
Research, 1, 209–215.

Halmi, K. A., Eckert, E., LaDu, T. J., &
Cohen, J. (1986). Anorexia nervosa.
Treatment efficacy of cyproheptadine
and amitriptyline. *Archives of General*
Psychiatry, 43, 177–181.

Halmi, K. A., Eckert, E., Marchi, P.,
Sampugnaro, V., Apple, R., & Cohen, J.
(1991). Comorbidity of psychiatric
diagnoses in anorexia nervosa. *Archives*
of General Psychiatry, 48, 712–718.

Hanefeld, M., & Sachse, G. (2002). The
effects of orlistat on body weight and
glycaemic control in overweight
patients with type 2 diabetes:
Randomized placebo-controlled trial.
Diabetes, Obesity, and Metabolism, 4,
415–423.

Hannum, S. M., Carson, L., Evans, E. M.,
Canene, K. A., Petr, E. L., Bui, L., et al.
(2004). Use of portion-controlled
entrees enhances weight loss in women.
Obesity Research, 12, 538–546.

Hanotin, C., Thomas, F., Jones, S. P.,
Leutenegger, E., & Drouin, P. (1998).
Efficacy and tolerability of sibutramine
in obese patients: A dose-ranging
study. *International Journal of Obesity and*
Related Metabolic Disorders, 22, 32–38.

Hasler, G., Pine, D. S., Gamma, A., Milos,
G., Ajdacic, V., Eich, D., et al. (2004).
The associations between
psychopathology and being
overweight: A 20-year prospective

study. *Psychological Medicine, 34,* 1047–
1057.

Hauner, H., Meier, M., Wendlan, G.,
Kurscheid, T., & Lauterbach, K. (2002).
Weight reduction by sibutramine in
obese subjects in primary care
medicine: The S.A.T. Study.
Experimental and Clinical Endocrinology
and Diabetes, 112, 201–207.

Hauptman, J., Lucas, C., Boldrin, M. N.,
Collins, H., & Segal, K. R. (2000).
Orlistat in the long-term treatment of
obesity in primary care settings.
Archives of Family Medicine, 9, 160–167.

Hay, P. J. (1998). The epidemiology of
eating disorder behaviors: An
Australian community-based survey.
International Journal of Eating Disorders,
23, 371–382.

Hay, P., Bacaltchuk, J., Claudino, A., Ben-
Tovim, D., & Yong, P. Y. (2003).
Individual psychotherapy in the
outpatient treatment of adults with
anorexia nervosa. *Cochrane Database of*
Systematic Reviews, 4, CD003909.

Hay, P. J., Bacaltchuk, J., & Stefano, S.
(2004). Psychotherapy for bulimia
nervosa and binging. *Cochrane Database*
Systematic Reviews, 1, CB000562.

Hay, P. J., Fairburn, C. G., & Doll, H. A.
(1996). The classification of bulimic
eating disorders: A community-based
cluster analysis study. *Psychological*
Medicine, 26, 801–812.

Heatherton, T. F., Nichols, P., Mahamedi,
F., & Keel, P. (1995). Body weight,
dieting, and eating disorder symptoms
among college students, 1982–1992.
American Journal of Psychiatry, 152,
1623–1629.

Hedley, A. A., Ogden, C. L., Johnson, C. L.,
Carroll, M. D., Curtin, L. R., & Flegal,
K. M. (2004). Prevalence of overweight
and obesity among US children,
adolescents, and adults, 1999–2002.
Journal of the American Medical
Association, 291, 2847–2850.

Heinssen, R. K., Levendusky, P. G., &

Hunter, R. H. (1995). Client as colleague: Therapeutic contracting with the seriously mentally ill. *American Psychologist, 50,* 522–532.

Helmrich, S. P., Ragland, D. R., Leung, R. W., Paffenbarger, R. S. (1991). Physical activity and reduced occurrence of non-insulin-dependent diabetes mellitus. *New England Journal of Medicine, 325,* 147–152.

Herpertz, S., Kielmann, R., Wolf, A. M., Hebebrand, J., & Senf, W. (2004). Do psychosocial variables predict weight loss or mental health after obesity surgery? A systematic review. *Obesity Research, 12,* 1554–1569.

Herpertz, S., Kielmann, R., Wolf, A. M., Langkafel, M., Senf, W., & Hebebrand, J. (2003). Does obesity surgery improve psychosocial functioning? A systematic review. *International Journal of Obesity & Related Metabolic Disorders, 27,* 1300–1314.

Herpertz, S., & Nielsen, S. (2003). Comorbidity of diabetes mellitus and eating disorders. In J. Treasure, U. Schmidt, & E. van Furth (Eds.), *Handbook of eating disorders.* Chichester: Wiley.

Herpertz, S., Wagener, R., Albus, C., Kocnar, M., Wagner, R., Best, F., et al. (1998). Diabetes mellitus and eating disorders: A multicenter study on the comorbidity of the two diseases. *Journal of Psychosomatic Research, 44,* 503–515.

Herpertz-Dahlmann, B., Muller, B., Herpertz, S., Heussen, N., Hebebrand, J., & Remschmidt, H. (2001). Prospective 10-year follow-up in adolescent anorexia nervosa: Course, outcome, psychiatric comorbidity, and psychosocial adaptation. *Journal of Child Psychology and Psychiatry and Allied Disciplines, 42,* 603–612.

Herzog, D. B., Dorer, D. J., Keel, P. K., Selwyn, S. E., Ekeblad, E. R., Flores, A. T., et al. (1999). Recovery and relapse in anorexia and bulimia nervosa: A 7.5-year follow-up study. *Journal of the American Academy of Child and Adolescent Psychiatry, 38,* 829–837.

Herzog, D. B., Hopkins, J. D., & Burns, C. D. (1993). A follow-up study of 33 subdiagnostic eating disordered women. *International Journal of Eating Disorders, 14,* 261–267.

Herzog, D. B., Keller, M. B., Lavori, P. W., & Ott, I. L. (1987). Social impairments in bulimia. *International Journal of Eating Disorders, 6,* 741–747.

Herzog, D. B., Keller, M. B., Sacks, N. R., Yeh, C. J., & Lavori, P. W. (1992). Psychiatric comorbidity in treatment-seeking anorexics and bulimics. *Journal of the American Academy of Child and Adolescent Psychiatry, 31,* 810–818.

Herzog, D. B., Nussbaum, K. M., & Marmor, A. K. (1996). Comorbidity and outcome in eating disorders. *Psychiatric Clinics of North America, 19,* 843–859.

Heshka, S., Anderson, J. W., Atkinson, R. L., Greenway, F. L., Hill, J. O., Phinney, S. D., et al. (2003). Weight loss and self-help compared with a structured commercial program: A randomized trial. *Journal of the American Medical Association, 289,* 1792–1798.

Heymsfield, S. B., van Mierlo, C. A. J., van der Knaap, H. C. M., Heo, M., & Frier, H. I. (2003). Weight management using a meal replacement strategy: Meta and pooling analysis from six studies. *International Journal of Obesity, 27,* 537–549.

Hickey, M. S., Pories, W. J., MacDonald, K. G., Cory, K. A., Dohm, G. L., Swanson, M. S., et al. (1998). A new paradigm for type 2 diabetes mellitus: Could it be a new disease of the foregut? *Annals of Surgery, 227,* 637–643.

Higgins, M., Kannel, W., Garrison, R., Pinsky, J., & Stokes, J., 3rd (1988). Hazards of obesity – the Framingham experience. *Acta Medica Scandinavica, 723,* 23–36.

Hill, A. J., & Silver, E. K. (1995). Fat

friendless and unhealthy: 9-year old children's perception of body shape stereotypes. *International Journal of Obesity and Related Metabolic Disorders, 19*, 423–430.

Hoek, H. W. (1991). The incidence and prevalence of anorexia nervosa and bulimia nervosa in primary care. *Psychological Medicine, 21*, 455–460.

Hoek, H. W. (1993). Review of the epidemiological studies of eating disorders. *International Review of Psychiatry, 5*, 61–74.

Hoek, H. W. (2002). Distribution of eating disorders. In C. G. Fairburn & K. D. Brownell (Eds.), *Eating disorders and obesity: A comprehensive handbook* (pp. 233–237). New York: Guilford Press.

Hoek, H. W., Bartelds, A. I. M., Bosveld, J. J. F., van der Graaf, Y., Limpens, V. E. L., Maiwald, M., et al. (1995). Impact of urbanization on detection rates of eating disorders. *American Journal of Psychiatry, 152*, 1272–1278.

Hoek, H. W., van Harten, P. N., Hermans, K. M., Katzman, M. A., Matroos, G. E., & Susser, E. S. (2005). The incidence of anorexia nervosa on Curacao. *American Journal of Psychiatry, 162*, 748–752.

Hoek, H. W., & van Hoeken, D. (2003). Review of the prevalence and incidence of eating disorders. *International Journal of Eating Disorders, 34*, 383–396.

Hollander, P. A., Elbein, S. C., Hirsch, I. B., Kelley, D., McGill, J., Taylor, T., et al. (1998). Role of orlistat in the treatment of obese patients with type 2 diabetes: A 1-year randomized double-blind study. *Diabetes Care, 21*, 1288–1294.

Howard, W. T., Evans, K. K., Quintero-Howard, C. V., Bowers, W. A., & Anderson, A. E. (1999). Predictors of success or failure of transition to day hospital treatment for inpatients with anorexia nervosa. *American Journal of Psychiatry, 156*, 1697–1702.

Hsu, L. K. G. (1990). *Eating disorders*. New York: Guilford Press.

Hu, F. B., Stampfer, M. J., Haffner, S. M., Solomon, C. G., Willett, W. C., & Manson, J. E. (2002). Elevated risk of cardiovascular disease prior to clinical diagnosis of type 2 diabetes. *Diabetes Care, 25*, 1129–1134.

Hudson, J. I., McElroy, S. L., Raymond, N. C., Crow, S., Keck, P. E. Jr., Carter, W. P., et al. (1998). Fluvoxamine treatment of binge eating disorder: A multicenter, placebo-controlled, double-blind trial. *American Journal of Psychiatry, 155*, 1756–1762.

Hudson, J. I., Pope, H. G., Jonas, J. M., & Yurgelun-Todd, D. (1983). Phenomenologic relationship of eating disorders to major affective disorder. *Psychiatry Research, 9*, 345–354.

Hughes, S. H., & Hughes, S. (2004). The female athlete syndrome: Anorexia nervosa – reflections on a personal journey. *Orthopaedic Nursing, 23*, 252–260.

Isomaa, B., Almgren, P., Tuomi, T., Forsen, B., Lahti, K., Nissen, M., et al. (2001). Cardiovascular morbidity and mortality associated with the metabolic syndrome. *Diabetes Care, 24*, 683–689.

Jakicic, J. M., Winters, C., Lang, W., & Wing, R. R. (1999). Effects of intermittent exercise and use of home exercise equipment on adherence, weight loss, and fitness in overweight women: A randomized trial. *Journal of the American Medical Association, 282*, 1554–1560.

Johnson, C., & Connors, M. (1987). *The etiology and treatment of eating disorders: A critical analysis*. New York: Basic Books.

Johnson, C. L., Stuckey, M. K., Lewis, L. D., & Schwartz, D. M. (1982). Bulimia: A descriptive study of 316 cases. *International Journal of Eating Disorders, 2*, 3–16.

Johnson, J. G., Spitzer, R. L., & Williams, J. B. W. (2001). Health problems, impairment and illnesses associated with bulimia nervosa and binge eating disorder among primary care and obstetric gynecology patients. *Psychological Medicine, 31*, 1455–1466.

Johnson, W. G., Kirk, A. A., & Reed, A. E. (2001). Adolescent version of the questionnaire of eating and weight patterns: Reliability and gender differences. *International Journal of Eating Disorders, 29*, 94–96.

Kalarchian, M. A., Wilson, G. T., Brolin, R. E., & Bradley, L. (2000). Assessment of eating disorders in bariatric surgery candidates: Self-report versus interview. *International Journal of Eating Disorders, 28*, 465–469.

Kanaley, J. A., Andresen-Reid, M. L., Oenning, L., Kottke, B. A., & Jensen, M. D. (1993). Differential health benefits of weight loss in upper-body and lower-body obese women. *American Journal of Clinical Nutrition, 57*, 20–26.

Kane, J. M., Quitkin, F., Rifkin, A., Wegner, J., Rosenberg, G., & Borenstein, M. (1983). Attitudinal changes of involuntarily committed patients following treatment. *Archives of General Psychiatry, 40*, 374–377.

Kaplan, A. S., & Olmsted, M. P. (1997). Partial hospitalization. In D. M. Garner & P. E. Garfinkel (Eds.), *Handbook of treatment for eating disorders* (2nd ed., pp. 354–360). New York: Guilford Press.

Katzman, M. A., Hermans, K. M., Van Hoeken, D., & Hoek, H. W. (2004). Not your "typical island woman": Anorexia nervosa is reported only in subcultures in Curacao. *Culture Medicine and Psychiatry, 28*, 463–492.

Kaya, A., Aydin, N., Topsever, P., Filiz, M., Ozturk, A., Dagar, A., et al. (2004). Efficacy of sibutramine, orlistat, and combination therapy on short-term weight management in obese patients. *Biomedicine and Pharmacotherapy, 58*, 582–587.

Kaye, W. H., Gwirtsman, H. E., George, D. T., Weiss, S. R., & Jimerson, D. C. (1986). Relationship of mood alterations to bingeing behaviour in bulimia. *British Journal of Psychiatry, 149*, 479–485.

Kaye, W. H., Lilenfeld, L. R., Plotnicov, K., Merikangis, K. R., Nagy, L., Strober, M., et al. (1996). Bulimia nervosa and substance dependence: Association and family transmission. *Alcohol Clinical and Experimental Research, 20*, 878–881.

Kaye, W. H., Nagata, T., Weltzin, T. E., Hsu, L. K., Sokol, M. S., McConaha, C., et al. (2001). Double-blind placebo-controlled administration of fluoxetine in restricting- and restricting-purging-type anorexia nervosa. *Biological Psychiatry, 49*, 644–652.

Kaye, W. H., Weltzin, T. E., McKee, M., McConaha, C., Hansen, D., & Hsu, L. K. (1992). Laboratory assessment of feeding behavior in bulimia nervosa and healthy women: Methods for developing a human-feeding laboratory. *American Journal of Clinical Nutrition, 55*, 372–380.

Keel, P. K., Crow, S., Davis, T. L., & Mitchell, J. E. (2002). Assessment of eating disorders: Comparison of interview and questionnaire data from a long-term follow-up study of bulimia nervosa. *Journal of Psychosomatic Research, 53*, 1043–1047.

Keel, P. K., Dorer, D. J., Eddy, K. T., Franko, D., Charatan, D. L., & Herzog, D. B. (2003). Predictors of mortality in eating disorders. *Archives of General Psychiatry, 60*, 179–183.

Keel, P. K., Fichter, M., Quadflieg, N., Bulik, C. M., Baxter, M. G., Thornton, L., et al. (2004). Application of a latent class analysis to empirically define eating disorder phenotypes. *Archives of General Psychiatry, 61*, 192–200.

Keel, P. K., Mayer, S. A., & Harnden-Fischer, J. H. (2001). Importance of size in defining binge eating episodes in bulimia nervosa. *International Journal of Eating Disorders, 29,* 294–301.

Keel, P. K., & Mitchell, J. E. (1997). Outcome in bulimia nervosa. *American Journal of Psychiatry, 154,* 313–321.

Keel, P. K., Mitchell, J. E., Miller, K. B., Davis, T. L, & Crow, S. J. (1999). Long-term outcome of bulimia nervosa. *Archives of General Psychiatry, 56,* 63–69.

Keith, S. W., Redden, D. T., Katzmarzyk, P., Boggiano, M. M., Hanlon, E. C., Benca, R. M., et al. (in press). Putative contributors to the secular increase in obesity: Exploring the roads less traveled. *International Journal of Obesity and Related Metabolic Disorders.*

Kelley, D. E., Bray, G. A., Pi-Sunyer, F. X., Klein, S., Hill, J., Miles, J., et al. (2002). Clinical efficacy of orlistat therapy in overweight and obese patients with insulin-treated type 2 diabetes: A 1-year randomized controlled trial. *Diabetes Care, 25,* 1033–1041.

Kenardy, J., Mensch, M., Bowen, K., Green, B., Walton, J., & Dalton, M. (2001). Disordered eating behaviours in women with Type 2 diabetes mellitus. *Eating Behaviors, 2,* 183–192.

Kenardy, J., Mensch, M., Bowen, K., Pearson, S. A. (1994). A comparison of eating behaviors in newly diagnosed NIDDM patients and case-matched control subjects. *Diabetes Care, 17,* 1197–1199.

Kendler, K. S., MacLean, C., Neale, M., Kessler, R., Heath, A., & Eaves, L. (1991). The genetic epidemiology of bulimia nervosa. *American Journal of Psychiatry, 148,* 1627–1637.

Keys, A., Brozek, K., Henschel, A., Mickelson, O., & Taylor, H. L. (1950). *The biology of human starvation.* Minneapolis: University of Minnesota Press.

Kirkley, B. G., Schneider, J. A., Agras, W. S., & Bachman, J. A. (1985). Comparison of two group treatments for bulimia.

Journal of Clinical and Consulting Psychology, 53, 43–48.

Kissileff, H. R., Walsh, B. T., Kral, J. G., & Cassidy, S. M. (1986). Laboratory studies of eating behavior in women with bulimia. *Physiological Behavior, 38,* 563–570.

Kjellin, L., Andersson, K., Candefjord, I. L., Palmstierna, T., & Wallsten, T. (1997). Ethical benefits and costs of coercion in short-term inpatient psychiatric care. *Psychiatric Services, 48,* 1567–1570.

Klesges, L. M., Estabrooks, P. A., Dzewaltowski, D. A., Bull, S. S., Glasgow, R. E. (2005). Beginning with the application in mind: Designing and planning health behavior change interventions to enhance dissemination. *Annals of Behavioral Medicine, 29,* 66–75.

Klump, K. L., & Gobrogge, K. L. (2005). A review and primer of molecular genetic studies of anorexia nervosa. *International Journal of Eating Disorders, 37,* S43–S48.

Klump, K. L., Wonderlich, S., Lehoux, P., Lilenfeld, L. R., & Bulik, C. M. (2002). Does environment matter? A review of nonshared environment and eating disorders. *International Journal of Eating Disorders, 31,* 118–135.

Kouba, S., Hallstrom, T., Lindholm, C., & Hirschberg, A. L. (2005). Pregnancy and neonatal outcomes in women with eating disorders. *Obstetrics and Gynecology, 105,* 255–260.

Kraig, K. A., & Keel, P. K. (2001). Weight-based stigmatization in children. *International Journal of Obesity, 25,* 1661–1666.

Kral, J. G., Brolin, R. E., Buchwald, H., Pories, W. J., Sarr, M. G., Sugerman, H. J., et al. (2002). Research considerations in obesity surgery. *Obesity Research, 10,* 63–64.

Kramer, F. M., Jeffery, R. W., Forster, J. L., & Snell, M. K. (1989). Long-term follow-up of behavioral treatment for obesity – patterns of weight regain among men and women. *International Journal of Obesity, 13,* 123–136.

Kripke, D. F., Garfinkel, L., Wingard, D. L., Klauber, M. R., & Maler, M. R. (2002). Mortality associated with sleep duration and insomnia. *Archives of General Psychiatry, 59,* 137–138.

Kruger, J., Galuska, D. A., Serdula, M. K., & Jones, D. A. (2004). Attempting to lose weight: Specific practices among U.S. adults. *American Journal of Preventative Medicine, 26,* 402–406.

Kuczmarski, R. J., Flegal, K. M., Campbell, S. M., & Johnson, C. L. (1994). Increasing prevalence of overweight among U.S. adults. The National Health and Nutrition Examination Surveys, 1963–1991. *Journal of the American Medical Association, 272,* 205–211.

Kurz, X., & Van Ermen, A. (1997). Valvular heart disease associated with fenfluramine-phentermine. *New England Journal of Medicine, 337,* 1772–1773.

Laederach-Hoffman, K., Graf, C., Horber, F., Lippuner, K., Lederer, S., Michel, R., et al. (1999). Imipramine and diet counseling with psychological support in the treatment of obese binge eaters: A randomized, placebo-controlled double-blind study. *International Journal of Eating Disorders, 26,* 231–244.

Latner, J. D., & Stunkard, A. J. (2003). Getting worse: The stigmatization of obese children. *Obesity Research, 11,* 452–456.

Latner, J. D., Wetzler, S., Goodman E. R., & Glinski, J. (2004). Gastric bypass in a low-income, inner-city population: Eating disturbances and weight loss. *Obesity Research, 12,* 956–961.

Lean, M. (1997). Sibutramin – a review of clinical efficacy. *International Journal of Obesity and Related Metabolic Disorders, 21,* S30–36.

Lee, C. D., Jackson, A. S., & Blair, S. N. (1998). US weight guidelines: Is it also important to consider cardiorespiratory fitness? *International Journal of Obesity and Related Metabolic Disorders, 22,* S2–S7.

Leitenberg, H., Rosen, J. C., Wolf, J., Vara, L. S., Detzer, M. J., & Srebnik, D. (1994). Comparison of cognitive behaviour therapy and desipramine in the treatment of bulimia nervosa. *Behaviour Research and Therapy, 32,* 37–45.

Levendusky, P. G., Willis, B. S., & Ghinassi, F. A. (1994). The therapeutic contracting program: A comprehensive continuum of care model. *Psychiatric Quarterly, 65,* 189–208.

Levine, J. A., Eberhardt, N. L., & Jensen, M. D. (1999). Role of nonexercise activity thermogenesis in resistance to fat gain in humans. *Science, 283,* 212–214.

Levine, J. A., Lanningham-Foster, L. M., McCrady, S. K., Krizan, A. C., Olson, L. R., Kane, P. H., et al. (2005). Interindividual variation in posture allocation: Possible role in human obesity. *Science, 307,* 584–586.

Lichtenbelt, W. V. M., & Fogelholm, M. (1992). Body composition. In M. D. Westererp-Planenga, A. B. Steffens, & A.Tremblay (Eds.), *Regulation of food intake and energy expenditure* (pp. 383–404). Milan: Medical Publishing and New Media.

Lichtman, S. W., Pirarska, K., Berman, E. R., Pestone, M., Dowling, H., Offenbacher, E., et al. (1992). Discrepency between self-reported and actual caloric intake and exercise in obese subjects. *New England Journal of Medicine, 327,* 1893–1898.

Lilenfeld, L. R., Kaye, W. H., Greeno, C. G., Merikangas, K. R., Plotnicov, K., Pollice, C., et al. (1998). A controlled family study of anorexia nervosa and bulimia nervosa: Psychiatric disorders in first-degree relatives and effects of proband comorbidity. *Archives of General Psychiatry, 55,* 603–610.

Lilenfeld, L. R., Stein, D., Bulik, C. M.,

Strober, M., Plotnicov, K., Pollice, C., et al. (2000). Personality traits among currently eating disordered, recovered, and never ill first-degree female relatives of bulimic and control women. *Psychological Medicine, 30,* 1399–1410.

Lock, J., Agras, W. S., Bryson, S., & Kraemer, H. C. (2005). A comparison of short- and long-term family therapy for adolescent anorexia nervosa. *Journal of the American Academy of Child and Adolescent Psychiatry, 44,* 632–639.

Lock, J., & Le Grange, D. (2001). Can family-based treatment of anorexia nervosa be manualized? *Journal of Psychotherapy Practice and Research, 10,* 253–261.

Lock, J., Le Grange, D., Agras, W. S., & Dare, C. (2001). *Treatment manual for anorexia nervosa: A family-based approach.* New York: Guilford Press.

Loeb, K. L., Wilson, G. T., Gilbert, J. S., & Labouvie, E. (2000). Guided and unguided self-help for binge eating. *Behaviour Research and Therapy, 38,* 259–272.

Loro, A. D., & Orleans, C. S. (1981). Binge eating in obesity: Preliminary findings and guidelines for behavioral analyses and treatment. *Addictive Behaviors, 6,* 155–166.

Lucas, A. R., Beard, C. M., O'Fallon, W. M., & Kurland, L. T. (1991). 50-year trends in the incidence of anorexia nervosa in Rochester, Minn: A population-based study. *American Journal of Psychiatry, 148,* 917–922.

Lucas, A. R., Crowson, C. S., O'Fallon, W. M., & Melton, L. J., 3rd. (1999). The ups and downs of anorexia nervosa. *International Journal of Eating Disorders, 26,* 397–405.

MacDonald, K. G. (2003). Overview of the epidemiology of obesity and the early histories of procedures to remedy morbid obesity. *Archives of Surgery, 138,* 357–360.

Mannucci, E., Rotella, F., Ricca, V., Moretti, S., Placidi, G. F., & Rotella, C. M. (2005). Eating disorders in patients with type 1 diabetes: A meta-analysis. *Journal of Endocrinological Investigation, 28,* 417–419.

Marcus, M. D., Wing, R. R., Ewing, L., Kern, E., McDermott, M., & Gooding, W. (1990). A double-blind, placebo-controlled trial of fluoxetine plus behavior modification in the treatment of obese binge-eaters and non-binge-eaters. *American Journal of Psychiatry, 147,* 876–881.

Marcus, M. D., Wing, R. R., & Hopkins, J. (1988). Obese binge eaters: Affect, cognitions, and response to behavioral weight control. *Journal of Consulting and Clinical Psychology, 56,* 433–439.

Masheb, R. M., & Grilo, C. M. (2000). Binge eating disorder: The need for additional diagnostic criteria. *Comprehensive Psychiatry, 41,* 159–162.

Masheb, R. M., & Grilo, C. M. (2002). Weight loss expectations in patients with binge-eating disorder. *Obesity Research, 10,* 309–314.

Masheb, R. M., & Grilo, C. M. (2002a). On the relation of flexible and rigid control of eating to body mass index and overeating in patients with eating disorder. *International Journal of Eating Disorders, 31,* 82–91.

Masheb, R. M., & Grilo, C. M. (2003). The nature of body image disturbance in patients with binge eating disorder. *International Journal of Eating Disorders, 33,* 333–341.

Masheb, R. M., & Grilo, C. M. (2006). Emotional overeating and its associations with eating disorder psychopathology among overweight patients with binge eating disorder. *International Journal of Eating Disorders, 39,* 141–146.

Mason, E. E., & Ito, C. (1967). Gastric bypass in obesity. *Surgical Clinics North America, 47,* 1345–1351.

McCann, U., & Agras, W. (1990).

Successful treatment of nonpurging bulimia nervosa with desipramine: A double-blind, placebo-controlled study. *American Journal of Psychiatry, 147,* 1509–1513.

McCann, U. D., Seiden, L. S., Rubin, L. J., & Ricaurte, G. A. (1997). Brain serotonin neurotoxicity and primary pulmonary hypertension from fenfluramine and dexfenfluramine. A systematic review of the evidence. *Journal of American Medical Association, 278,* 666–672.

McElroy, S. L., Arnold, L. M., Shapira, N. A., Keck, P. E. Jr., Rosenthal, N. R., Karim, M. R., et al. (2003a). Topiramate in the treatment of binge eating disorder associated with obesity: A randomized placebo-controlled trial. *American Journal of Psychiatry, 160,* 255–261.

McElroy, S. L., Casuto, L. S., Nelson, E. B., et al. (2000). Placebo-controlled trial of sertaline in the treatment of binge eating disorder. *American Journal of Psychiatry, 157,* 1004–1006.

McElroy, S. L., Hudson, J. I., Malhotra, S., Welge, J. A., Nelson, E. B., & Keck, P. E. Jr. (2003b). Citalopram in the treatment of binge-eating disorder: A placebo-controlled trial. *Journal of Clinical Psychiatry, 64,* 807–813.

McElroy, S. L., Shapira, N. A., Arnold, L. M., Keck, P. E., Rosenthal, N. R., Wu, S. C., et al. (2004). Topiramate in the long-term treatment of binge-eating disorder associated with obesity. *Journal of Clinical Psychiatry, 65,* 643–649.

McGlynn, E. A., Asch, S. M., Adams, J., et al. (2003). The quality of health care delivered to adults in the United States. *New England Journal of Medicine, 348,* 2635–2645.

McIntosh, V. V., Jordan, J., Carter, F. A., Luty, S. E., McKenzie, J. M., Bulik, C. M., et al. (2005). Three psychotherapies for anorexia nervosa: A randomized, controlled trial. *American Journal of Psychiatry, 162,* 741–747.

McKenzie, D. C., Johnson, R. K., Harvey-Berino, J., & Gold, B. C. (2002). Impact of interviewer's body mass index on under-representing energy intake in overweight and obese women. *Obesity Research, 10,* 471–477.

McMaster, R., Beale, B., Hillege, S., & Nagy, S. (2004). The parent experience of eating disorders: Interactions with health professionals. *International Journal of Mental Health Nursing, 13,* 67–73.

Meads, C., Gold, I., & Burls, A. (2001). How effective is outpatient care compared to inpatient care for the treatment of anorexia nervosa? A systematic review. *European Eating Disorders Review, 9,* 229–241.

Miles, J. M., Leiter, L., Hollander, P., Wadden, T., Anderson, J. W., Doyle, M., et al. (2002). Effect of orlistat in overweight and obese patients with type 2 diabetes treated with metformin. *Diabetes Care, 25,* 1123–1128.

Milos, G., Spindler, A., Schnyder, U., & Fairburn, C. G. (2005). Instability of the eating disorder diagnoses: A prospective study. *British Journal of Psychiatry, 187,* 573–578.

Mitchell, J. E., Fletcher, L., Hanson, K., Mussell, M. P., Seim, H., Crosby, R., et al. (2001). The relative efficacy of fluoxetine and manual-based self-help in the treatments of outpatients with bulimia nervosa. *Journal of Clinical Psychopharmacology, 21,* 298–304.

Mitchell, J. E., Mussell, M. P., Peterson, C. B., Crow S., Wonderlich, S. A., Crosby R. D., et al. (1999). Hedonics of binge eating in women with bulimia nervosa and binge eating disorder. *International Journal of Eating Disorders, 26,* 165–170.

Mitchell, J. E., & Peterson, C. (Eds.). (2005). *The assessment of patients with eating disorders.* New York: Guilford Press.

Mitchell, J. E., Pyle, R. L., & Eckert, E. D. (1981). Frequency and duration of binge-eating episodes in patients with bulimia. *American Journal of Psychiatry, 138* (6), 835–836.

Mitchell, J. E., Pyle, R. L., Eckert, E. D., Hatsukami, D., Pomeroy, C., & Zimmerman, R. (1990). A comparison study of antidepressants and structured intensive group therapy in the treatment of bulimia nervosa. *Archives of General Psychiatry, 471,* 49–157.

Mitka, M. (2003). Surgery for obesity – demand soars amid scientific, ethical questions. *Journal of the American Medical Association, 289,* 1761–1762.

Mizes, J. S., & Sloan, D. M. (1998). An empirical analysis of eating disorder, not otherwise specified: Preliminary support for a distinct subgroup. *International Journal of Eating Disorders, 23,* 233–242.

Mond, J. M., Hay, P. J., Rodgers, B., Owen, C., & Beumont, P. J. V. (2004). Validity of the Eating Disorder Examination Questionnaire (EDE-Q) in screening for eating disorders in community samples. *Behavior Research and Therapy, 42,* 551–567.

Morgan, H. G. (1977). Fasting girls and our attitudes to them. *British Medical Journal, 2*(6103), 1652–1655.

Mrdjenovic, G., & Levitsky, D. A. (2005). Children eat what they are served: The imprecise regulation of energy intake. *Appetite, 44,* 273–282.

Mussell, M. P., Mitchell, J. E., Weller, C. L., Raymond, N. C., Crow, S. J., & Crosby, R. (1995). Onset of binge eating, dieting, obesity, and mood disorders among subjects seeking treatment for binge eating disorder. *International Journal of Eating Disorders, 17,* 395–401.

National Cholesterol Education Program (NCEP, 2001). Executive summary of the third report of the NCEP Expert Panel on Detection, Evaluation, and Treatment of High Blood Cholesterol in Adults (Adult Treatment Panel III). *Journal of the American Medical Association, 285,* 2486–2497.

National Institute for Clinical Excellence (NICE, 2001/2004). *Guidance on the use of sibutramine for the treatment of obesity in adults.* NICE Clinical Guideline No. 31. London: National Institute for Clinical Excellence.

National Institute for Clinical Excellence (NICE, 2004). *Eating disorders – core interventions in the treatment and management of anorexia nervosa, bulimia nervosa, related eating disorders.* NICE Clinical Guideline No. 9. London: National Institute for Clinical Excellence.

National Institutes of Health (NIH, 1992). Gasterointestinal surgery for severe obesity: National Institute of Health Consensus Development Conference Statement. *American Journal of Clinical Nutrition, 55,* S615–S619.

National Institutes of Health, & National Heart, Lung, and Blood Institute (NHLBI, 1998a). *Obesity education initiative: Clinical guidelines on the identification, evaluation, and treatment of overweight and obesity in adults.* Washington, DC: U.S. Department Health Human Services.

National Institutes of Health, & National Heart, Lung, and Blood Institute (NHLBI, 1998b). Clinical guidelines on the identification, evaluation, and treatment of overweight and obesity in adults: executive summary. Expert Panel on the Identification, Evaluation, and Treatment of Overweight in Adults. *American Journal of Clinical Nutrition, 68,* 899–917.

National Institutes of Health, & National Heart, Lung, and Blood Institute (NHLBI, 1998c). Clinical guidelines on the identification, evaluation, and treatment of overweight and obesity in adults – the evidence report. *Obesity Research, 6,* 1S–209S.

National Task Force on the Prevention and

Treatment of Obesity (NFT, 2000a). Overweight, obesity, and health risk. *Archives of Internal Medicine, 160,* 898–904.

National Task Force on the Prevention and Treatment of Obesity (NFT, 2000b). Dieting and the development of eating disorders in overweight and obese adults. *Archives of Internal Medicine, 160,* 2581–2589.

Nauta, H., Hospers, H., Gerjo, K., & Jansen, A. (2000). A comparison between a cognitive and a behavioral treatment for obese binge eaters and obese non-binge eaters. *Behavior Therapy, 31,* 441–461.

Neumarker-Sztainer, D., Croll, J., Story, M., Hannan, P. J., French, S. A., & Perry, C. (2002a). Ethnic/racial differences in weight-related concerns and behaviors among adolescent girls and boys: Findings from Project EAT. *Journal of Psychosomatic Research, 53,* 963–974.

Neumarker-Sztainer, D., Jeffery, R. W., & French, S. A. (1997). Self-reported dieting: How should we ask? What does it mean? Associations between dieting and reported energy intake. *International Journal of Eating Disorders, 22,* 437–449.

Neumarker-Sztainer, D., Story, M., Hannan, P. J., Perry, C., & Irving, L. M. (2002b). Weight-related concerns and behaviors among overweight and nonoverweight adolescents: Implications for preventing weight-related disorders. *Archives of Pediatric and Adolescent Medicine, 156,* 171–178.

Nielsen, S. J., & Popkin, B. M. (2003). Patterns and trends in food portion sizes, 1977–1998. *Journal of the American Medical Association, 289,* 450–453.

Oeppen, J., & Vaupel, J. (2002). Broken limits to life expectancy. *Science, 296,* 1029–1031.

Ogden, C. L., Troiano, R. P., Briefel, R. R., Kuczmarski, R. J., Flegal, K. M., & Johnson, C. L. (1997). Prevalence of overweight among preschool children in the United States, 1971 through 1994. *Pediatrics, 99,* E1.

Olshansky, S. J., Passaro, D. J., Hershow, R. C., Layden, J., Carnes, B. A., Brody, J., et al. (2005). A potential decline in life expectancy in the United States in the 21st century. *New England Journal of Medicine, 352,* 1138–1145.

Olson, C. L., Schumaker, H. D., & Yawn, B. P. (1994). Overweight women delay medical care. *Archives of Family Medicine, 3,* 888–892.

O'Meara, S., Riemsma, R., Shirran, L., Mather, L., & ter Riet, G. (2002). The clinical effectiveness and cost-effectiveness of sibutramine in the management of obesity: A technology assessment. *Health Technology Assessment, 6,* 1–97.

O'Meara, S., Riemsma, R., Shirran, L., Mather, L., & ter Riet, G. (2004). A systematic review of the clinical effectiveness of orlistat used for the management of obesity. *Obesity Reviews, 5,* 51–68.

O'Reardon, J. P., Ringel, B. L., Dinges, D. F., Allison, K. C., Rogers, N., L., Martino, N. S., et al. (2004). Circadian eating and sleeping patterns of the night eating syndrome. *Obesity Research, 12,* 1789–1796.

Orvaschel, H., & Puig-Antich, J. (1987). *Schedule for affective disorder and schizophrenia for school-age children (version 4).* Pittsburgh: Western Psychiatric Institute and Clinic.

Paeratakul, S., White, M. A., Williamson, D. A., Ryan, D. H., & Bray, G. A. (2002). Sex, race/ethnicity, socioeconomic status, and BMI in relation to self-perception of overweight. *Obesity Research, 10,* 345–350.

Palmer, R. L., Birchall, H., McGrain, L., & Sullivan, V. (2002). Self-help for bulimic disorders: A randomized controlled trial comparing minimal guidance with face-to-face or telephone guidance.

British Journal of Psychiatry, 181, 230–235.

Parry-Jones, B., & Parry-Jones W. L. (1991). Bulimia: An archival review of its history in psychosomatic medicine. *International Journal of Eating Disorders, 10,* 129–143.

Passi, V. A., Bryson, S. W., & Lock, J. (2003). Assessment of eating disorders in adolescents with anorexia nervosa: Self-report questionnaire versus interview. *International Journal of Eating Disorders, 33,* 45–54.

Pate, R. R., Pratt, M., Blair, S. N., Haskell, W.L, Macera, C. A., Bouchard, C., et al. (1995). Physical activity and public health. A recommendation from the Centers for Disease Control and Prevention and the American College of Sports Medicine. *Journal of the American Medical Association, 273,* 402–407.

Patel, S. R., Ayas, N. T., Malhotra, M. R., White, D. P., Schernhammer, E. S., Speizer, F. E., et al. (2004). A prospective study of sleep duration and mortality risk in women. *Sleep, 27,* 440–444.

Pavlou, K. N., Krey, S., & Steffee, W. P. (1989). Exercise as an adjunct to weight loss and maintenance in moderately obese subjects. *American Journal of Clinical Nutrition, 49,* 1115–1123.

Peeters, A., Bonneux, L., Barendregt, J., & Nusselder, W. (2003). Methods of estimating years of life lost due to obesity. *Journal of the American Medical Association, 289,* 2941.

Penas-Lledo, E., Vaz Leal, F. J., & Waller, G. (2002). Excessive exercise in anorexia nervosa and bulimia nervosa: Relation to eating characteristics and general psychopathology. *International Journal of Eating Disorders, 31,* 370–375.

Pereira, M. A., Kartashov, A. I., Ebbeling, C. B., Van Horn, L., Slattery, M. L., Jacobs, D. R., et al. (2005). Fast-food habits, weight gain, and insulin resistance (the CARDIA study): 15-year prospective analysis. *Lancet, 365,* 36–42.

Perkins, S., Winn, S., Murray, J., Murphy, R., & Schmidt, U. (2004). A qualitative study of the experience of caring for a person with bulimia nervosa. Part 1: the emotional impact of caring. *International Journal of Eating Disorders, 36,* 256–268.

Perri, M. G., Martin, A. D., Leermakers, E. A., Sears, S. F., & Notelovitz, M. (1997). Effects of group- versus home-based exercise in the treatment of obesity. *Journal of Consulting and Clinical Psychology, 65,* 278–285.

Perri, M. G., McAllister, D. A., Gange, J. J., Jordan, R. C., McAdoo, W. G., & Nezu, A. M. (1988). Effects of four maintenance programs on the long-term management of obesity. *Journal of Consulting and Clinical Psychology, 56,* 529–534.

Perrin, E. M., Flower, K. B., & Ammerman, A. S. (2005). Pediatricians' own weight: Self perception, misclassification, and ease of counseling. *Obesity Research, 13,* 326–332.

Perusse, L., Rankinen, T., Zuberi, A., Chagnon, Y. C., Weisnagel, S. J., Argyropoulos, G., et al. (2005). The human obesity gene map: The 2004 update. *Obesity Research, 13,* 381–490.

Peterson, C. B., Mitchell, J. E., Engbloom, S., Nugent, S., Mussell, M. P., & Miller, J. P. (1998). Group cognitive-behavioral treatment of binge eating disorder: A comparison of therapist-led versus self-help formats. *International Journal of Eating Disorders, 24,* 125–136.

Peterson, C. B., Mitchell, J. E., Engbloom, S., Nugent, S., Pederson Mussell, M., Crow, S. J., et al. (2001). Self-help versus therapist-led group cognitive behavioral treatment of binge eating disorder at follow-up. *International Journal of Eating Disorders, 30,* 363–374.

Petro, A. E., Cotter, J., Cooper, D. A., Peters, J. C., Surwit, S. J., & Surwit, R. S. (2004). Fat, carbohydrate, and calories in the development of diabetes and obesity in the mouse. *Metabolism, 53,* 454–457.

Pike, K. M., Dohm, F. A., Striegel-Moore, R. H., Wilfley, D. E., & Fairburn, C. G. (2001). A comparison of black and white women with binge eating disorder. *American Journal of Psychiatry, 158,* 1455–1460.

Pine, D. S., Cohen, P., Brook, J., et al. (1997). Psychiatric symptoms in adolescence as predictors of obesity in early adulthood: A longitudinal study. *American Journal of Public Health, 97,* 1303–1310.

Pinhas-Hamiel, O., Dolan, L. M., Daniels, S. R., Standiford, D., Khoury, R. P., & Zeitler, P. (1996). Increased incidence of non-insulin dependent diabetes mellitus among adolescents. *Journal of Pediatrics, 12,* 608–615.

Pomeroy, C., & Mitchell, J. (1996). Medical complications and management of eating disorders. *Psychiatric Annals, 19,* 488–493.

Pope, G. D., Birkmeyer, J. D., & Finlayson, S. R. G. (2002). National trends in utilization and in-hospital outcomes of bariatric surgery. *Journal of Gastrointestinal Surgery, 6,* 855–860.

Pories, W. J., Swanson, M. S., MacDonald, K. G., Long, S. B., Morris, P. G., Brown, B. M., et al. (1995). Who would have thought it – an operation proves to be the most effective therapy for adult-onset diabetes-mellitus. *Annals of Surgery, 222,* 339–352.

Porzelius, L. K., Houston, C., Smith, M., Arfken, C., & Fisher, E. (1995). Comparison of a standard behavioral weight loss treatment and a binge eating weight loss treatment. *Behavior Therapy, 26,* 119–134.

Poston, W. S. C., Haddock, C. K., Pinkston, M. M., Pace, P., Karakoc, N. D., Reeves, R. S., et al. (2005). Weight loss with meal replacement plus snacks: A

randomized trial. *International Journal of Obesity, 29,* 1107–1114.

Potter, M. B., Vu, J. D., & Croughan-Minihane, M. (2001). Weight management: What patients want from their primary care physicians. *Journal of Family Practice, 50,* 513–518.

Power, C., & Jefferis, B. J. (2002). Fetal environment and subsequent obesity: A study of maternal smoking. *International Journal of Epidemiology, 31,* 413–419.

Pratt, E. M., Niego, S. H., & Agras, W. S. (1998). Does the size of a binge matter? *International Journal of Eating Disorders, 24,* 307–312.

Pryor, T., Wiederman, M. W., & McGilley, B. (1996). Laxative abuse among women with eating disorders: An indication of psychopathology. *International Journal of Eating Disorders, 20,* 13–18.

Pyle, R. L., Mitchell, J. E., & Eckert, E. D. (1981). Bulimia: A report of 34 cases. *Journal of Clinical Psychiatry, 42,* 60–64.

Quadflieg, N., & Fichter, M. M. (2003). The course and outcome of bulimia nervosa. *European Child and Adolescent Psychiatry, 12,* I99–109.

Ramsay, R., Ward, A., Treasure J., & Russell, G. F. (1999). Compulsory treatment in anorexia nervosa. Short-term benefits and long-term mortality. *British Journal of Psychiatry, 175,* 147–153.

Rand, C. S., & MacGregor, A. M. (1994). Adolescents having obesity surgery: A 6-year follow-up. *Southern Medical Journal, 87,* 1208–1213.

Rand, C. S. W., MacGregor, M. D., & Stunkard, A. J. (1997). The night eating syndrome in the general population and among post-operative obesity surgery patients. *International Journal of Eating Disorders, 22,* 65–69.

Ravussin, E., Valencia, M. E., Esparza, J., Bennett, P. H., & Schulz, L. O. (1994). Effects of a traditional lifestyle on obesity in Pima Indians. *Diabetes Care, 9,* 1067–1074.

Reas, D. L., Grilo, C. M., & Masheb, R. M. (2006). Reliability of the Eating Disorder Examination Questionnaire in patients with binge eating disorder. *Behaviour Research and Therapy, 44,* 43–51.

Reas, D. L., Masheb, R. M., & Grilo, C. M. (2004). Appearance versus health reasons for seeking treatment among obese patients with binge eating disorder. *Obesity Research, 12,* 758–760.

Reas, D. L., Schoemaker, C., Zipfel, S., & Williamson, D. A. (2001). Prognostic value of duration of illness and early intervention in bulimia nervosa: A systematic review of the outcome literature. *International Journal of Eating Disorders, 30,* 1–10.

Reas, D. L., Williamson, D. A., Martin, C. K., & Zucker, N. L. (2000). Duration of illness predicts outcome for bulimia nervosa: A long-term follow-up study. *International Journal of Eating Disorders, 27,* 428–434.

Rexrode, K. M., Carey, V. J., Hennekens, C. H., Walters, E. E., Colditz, G. A., Stampfer, M. J., et al. (1998). Abdominal adiposity and coronary heart disease in women. *Journal of the American Medical Association, 280,* 1843–1848.

Ricca, V., Mannucci, E., Mezzani, B., Di Bernardo, M., Zucchi, T., Paionni, A., et al. (2001). Psychopathological and clinical features of outpatients with an eating disorder not otherwise specified. *Eating and Weight Disorders, 6,* 157–165.

Richardson, H. B. (1946). Obesity as a manifestation of neurosis. *Medical Clinics of North America, 30,* 1187–1202.

Richardson, L. P., Davis, R., Poulton, R., et al. (2003). A longitudinal evaluation of adolescent depression and adult obesity. *Archives of Pediatric and Adolescent Medicine, 157,* 739–745.

Rippe, J. M., Ward, A., Porcari, J. P., & Freedson, P. S. (1988). Walking for health and fitness. *Journal of American Medical Association, 259,* 2720–2724.

Robb, A. S., Silber, T. J., Orrell-Valente, J. K., Valadez-Meltzer, A., Ellis, N., Dadson, M. J., et al. (2002). Supplemental nocturnal nasogastric refeeding for better short-term outcome in hospitalized adolescent girls with anorexia nervosa. *American Journal of Psychiatry, 159,* 1347–1353.

Robin, A. L., Siegel, P. T., Koepke, T., Moye, A. W., & Tice, S. (1994). Family therapy versus individual therapy for adolescent females with anorexia nervosa. *Journal of Developmental and Behavioral Pediatrics, 15,* 111–116.

Robin, A. L., Siegel, P. T., Moye, A. W., Gilroy, M., Dennis, A. B., & Sikand, A. (1999). A controlled comparison of family versus individual therapy for adolescents with anorexia nervosa. *Journal of the American Academy of Child and Adolescent Psychiatry, 38,* 1482–1489.

Rodin, J., Silberstein, L. R., & Striegel-Moore, R. H. (1985). Women and weight: A normative discontent. In T. B. Sonderegger (ed.), *Nebraska symposium on motivation* (pp. 267–308). Lincoln: University of Nebraska Press.

Rosen, J. C., Leitenberg, H., Fisher, C., & Khazam, C. (1986). Binge-eating episodes in bulimia nervosa: The amount and type of food consumed. *International Journal of Eating Disorders, 5,* 255–267.

Rossiter, E., & Agras, S. (1990). An empirical test of the DSM-III-R definition of binge. *International Journal of Eating Disorders, 9,* 513–518.

Russell, G. F. M. (1979). Bulimia nervosa: An ominous variant of anorexia nervosa. *Psychological Medicine, 9,* 429–448.

Russell, G. F. (2001). Involuntary treatment in anorexia nervosa. *Psychiatric Clinics North America, 24,* 337–349.

Russell, G. F. M., Szmulker, G. I., Dare, C., & Eisler, I. (1987). An evaluation of family therapy in anorexia nervosa and bulimia nervosa. *Archives of General Psychiatry, 44,* 1047–1056.

Samaha, F. F., Iqbal, N., Seshadri, P., Chicano, K. L., Daily, D. A., McGrory, J., et al. (2003). A low-carbohydrate as compared with a low-fat diet in severe obesity. *New England Journal of Medicine, 348,* 2074–2081.

Sampalis, J. S., Liberman, M., Auger, S., & Christou, N. V. (2004). The impact of weight reduction surgery on health-care costs in morbidly obese patients. *Obesity Surgery, 14,* 939–947.

Santonastaso, P., Saccon, D., & Favaro, A. (1997). Burden and psychiatric symptoms on key relatives of patients with eating disorders: A preliminary study. *Eating and Weight Disorders, 2,* 44–48.

Sari, R., Balci, M. K., Cakir, M., Altunbas, H., & Karayalcin, U. (2004). Comparison of efficacy of sibutramine or orlistat versus their combination in obese women. *Endocrine Research, 30,* 159–167.

Scagliusi, F. B., Polacow, V. O., Artioli, G. G., Benatti, F. B., & Lancha, A. H. Jr. (2003). Selective underreporting of energy intake in women: Magnitude, determinants, and effect of training. *Journal of the American Dietetic Association, 103,* 1306–1313.

Schauer, P. R., Burguera, B., Ikramuddin, S., Cottam, D., Gourash, W., Hamad, G., et al. (2003). Effect of laparoscopic Roux-en Y gastric bypass on type 2 diabetes mellitus. *Annals of Surgery, 238,* 467–484.

Schenck, C. H., & Mahowald, M. W. (1994). Review of nocturnal sleep-related eating disorders. *International Journal of Eating Disorders, 15,* 343–356.

Schmitz, K. H., Jacobs, D. R., Leon, A. S., Schreiner, P. J., & Sternfeld, B. (2000). Physical activity and body weight: Associations over ten years in the CARDIA study. *International Journal of Obesity and Related Metabolic Disorders, 24,* 1475–1487.

Schoken, D., Holloway, J. D., & Powers, P. (1989). Weight loss and the heart: Effects of anorexia nervosa and starvation. *Archives of Internal Medicine, 149,* 877–881.

Schwalberg, M. D., Barlow, D. H., Alger, S. A., & Howard, L. J. (1992). Comparison of bulimics, obese binge eaters, social phobics, and individuals with panic disorder on comorbidity across DSM-III-R anxiety disorders. *Journal of Abnormal Psychology, 101,* 675–681.

Schwartz, M. B., Chambliss, H. O, Brownell, K. D., Blair, S. N., & Billington, C. (2003). Weight bias among health professionals specializing in obesity. *Obesity Research, 11,* 1033–1039.

Serdula, M. K., Mokdad, A. H., Williamson, D. F., Galuska, D. A., Mendlein, J. M., & Heath, G. W. (1999). Prevalence of attempting weight loss and strategies for controlling weight. *Journal of the American Medical Association, 13,* 1353–1358.

Sharp, C. W., & Freeman, C. P. L. (1993). The medical complications of anorexia nervosa. *British Journal of Psychiatry, 162,* 452–462.

Sherwood, N. E., Jeffery, R. W., & Wing, R. R. (1999). Binge status as a predictor of weight loss treatment outcome. *International Journal of Obesity, 23,* 485–493.

Sjostrom, C. D., Lissner, L., Wedel, H., & Sjostrom, L. (1999). Reduction in incidence of diabetes, hypertension and lipid disturbances after intentional weight loss induced by bariatric surgery: The SOS Intervention Study. *Obesity Research, 7,* 477–484.

Sjostrom, C. D., Peltonen, M., Wedel, H., & Sjostrom, L. (2000). Differentiated long-term effects of intentional weight loss on diabetes and hypertension. *Hypertension, 36,* 20–25.

Sjostrom, L., Lindroos, A. K., Peltonen, M., Torgerson, J., Bouchard, C., Carlsson, B., et al. (2004). Lifestyle, diabetes, and cardiovascular risk factors 10 years after bariatric surgery. *New England Journal of Medicine, 351,* 2683–2693.

Sjostrom, L., Rissanen, A., Andersen, T., Boldrin, M., Golay, A., Koppeschaar, H. P., et al. (1998). Randomized placebo-controlled trial of orlistat for weight loss and prevention of weight regain in obese patients. European Multicentre Orlistat Study Group. *Lancet, 352,* 167–172.

Sloan, D. M., Mizes, J. S., & Epstein, E. M. (2005). Empirical classification of eating disorders. *Eating Behaviors, 6,* 53–62.

Smith, C. J., Nelson, R. G., Hardy, S. A., Manahan, E. M., Bennett, P. H., & Knowler, W. C. (1996). Survey of the diet of Pima Indians using quantitative food frequency assessment and 24-hour recall. *Journal of the American Dietetics Association, 96,* 778–784.

Smith, D. E., & Wing, R. R. (1991). Diminished weight loss and behavioral compliance during repeated diets in obese patients with type II diabetes. *Health Psychology, 10,* 378–383.

Smith, I. G., & Goulder, M. A. (2001). Randomized placebo-controlled trial of long-term treatment with sibutramine in mild to moderate obesity. *Journal of Family Practice, 50,* 505–512.

Sorbara, M., & Geliebter, A. (2002). Body image disturbance in obese outpatients before and after weight loss in relation to race, gender, binge eating, and age of onset of obesity. *International Journal of Eating Disorders, 31,* 416–423.

Soundy, T. J., Lucas, A. R., Suman, V. J., & Melton, L. J., 3rd (1995). Bulimia nervosa in Rochester, Minnesota from 1980–1990. *Psychological Medicine, 25,* 1065–1071.

Spitzer, R. L., Devlin, M. J., Walsh, B. T., Hasin, D., Wing, R. R., Marcus, M. D., et al. (1992). Binge eating disorder: A multisite field trial for the diagnostic criteria. *International Journal of Eating Disorders, 11,* 191–203.

Spitzer, R. L., Yanovski, S., Wadden, T., Wing, R., Marcus, M. D., Stunkard, A., et al. (1993). Binge eating disorder: Its further validation in a multisite study. *International Journal of Eating Disorders, 13,* 137–153.

Spurrell, E. B., Wilfley, D. E., Tanofsky, M. B., & Brownell, K. D. (1997). Age of onset for binge eating: Are there different pathways to binge eating? *International Journal of Eating Disorders, 21,* 55–65.

Stamler, J., Wentworth, D., & Neaton, J. D. (1986). Is relationship between serum cholesterol and risk of premature death from coronary disease continuous or graded? Findings in 356, 222 primary screenees of the Multiple Risk Factor Intervention Trial (MRFIT). *Journal of the American Medical Association, 256,* 2823–2828.

Stein, D. M., & Laakso, W. (1988). Bulimia: A historical perspective. *International Journal of Eating Disorders, 7,* 201–210.

Steinhausen, H. C. (2002). The outcome of anorexia nervosa in the 20th century. *American Journal of Psychiatry, 159,* 1284–1293.

Stern, L., Iqbal, N., Seshadri, P., Chicano, K. L., Daily, D. A., McGrory, J., et al. (2004). The effects of low-carbohydrate versus conventional weight loss diets in severely obese adults: One-year follow-up of a randomized trial. *Annals of Internal Medicine, 140,* 778–785.

Stice, E., & Agras, W. S. (1999). Subtyping bulimic women along dietary restraint and negative affect dimensions. *Journal of Consulting and Clinical Psychology, 67,* 460–469.

Stice, E., Agras, W. S., Telch, C., Halmi, K. A., Mitchell, J. E., & Wilson, G. T. (2001). Subtyping binge eating disordered women along dieting and negative affect dimensions. *International Journal of Eating Disorders, 30*, 11–27.

Stirn, A., Overbeck, G., & Pokorny, D. (2005). The core conflictual relationship theme (CCRT) applied to literary works: An analysis of two novels written by authors suffering from anorexia nervosa. *International Journal of Eating Disorders, 38*, 147–156.

Stock, S. L., Goldberg, E., Corbett, S., & Katzman, D. K. (2002). Substance use in female adolescents with eating disorders. *Journal of Adolescent Health, 31*, 176–182.

Strauss, R. S., Bradley, L. J., & Brolin, R. E. (2001). Gastric bypass surgery in adolescents with morbid obesity. *Journal of Pediatrics, 138*, 499–504.

Striegel-Moore, R. H., Dohm, F. A., Solomon, E. E., Fairburn, C. G., Pike, K. M., & Wilfley, D. E. (2000a). Subthreshold binge eating disorder. *International Journal of Eating Disorders, 27*, 270–278.

Striegel-Moore, R. H., Dohm, F. A., Wilfley, D. E., Pike, K. M., Bray, N. L., Kraemer, H. C., et al. (2004). Toward an understanding of health services use in women with binge eating disorder. *Obesity Research, 12*, 799–806.

Striegel-Moore, R. H., & Franko, D. L. (2003). Epidemiology of binge eating disorder. *International Journal of Eating Disorders, 34*, 19–29.

Striegel-Moore, R. H., Silberstein, L. R., & Rodin, J. (1993). The social self in bulimia nervosa: Public self-consciousness, social anxiety, and perceived fraudulence. *Journal of Abnormal Psychology, 102*, 297–303.

Striegel-Moore, R. H., Wilfley, D. E., Pike, K. M., Dohm, F., & Fairburn, C. G. (2000b). Recurrent binge eating in black American women. *Archives of Family Medicine, 9*, 83–87.

Striegel-Moore, R. H., Wilson, G. T., Wilfley, D. E., Elder, K. A., & Brownell, K. D. (1998). Binge eating in an obese community sample. *International Journal of Eating Disorders, 23*, 27–37.

Strober, M. (2004). Managing the chronic, treatment-resistant patient with anorexia nervosa. *International Journal of Eating Disorders, 36*, 245–255.

Strober, M., Freeman, R., Lampert, C., Diamond, J., & Kaye, W. (2000). Controlled family study of anorexia nervosa and bulimia nervosa: Evidence of shared liability and transmission of partial syndromes. *American Journal of Psychiatry, 157*, 393–401.

Strober, M., Freeman, R., & Morrell, W. (1997). The long-term course of severe anorexia nervosa in adolescents: Survival analysis of recovery, relapse, and outcome predictors over 10–15 years in a prospective study. *International Journal of Eating Disorders, 22*, 339–360.

Stuart, R. R. (1967). Behavioral control of overeating. *Behaviour Research and Therapy, 5*, 357–365.

Stunkard, A. J. (1959). Eating patterns and obesity. *Psychiatric Quarterly, 33*, 284–295.

Stunkard, A. J., Berkowitz, R., Tanrikut, C., Reiss, E., & Young, L. (1996a). d-Fenfluramine treatment of binge eating disorder. *American Journal of Psychiatry, 153*, 1455–1459.

Stunkard, A. J., Berkowitz, R., Wadden, T., Tanrikut, C., Reiss, E., & Young, L. (1996b). Binge eating disorder and the night eating syndrome. *International Journal of Obesity and Related Metabolic Disorders, 20*, 1–6.

Stunkard, A. J., Grace, W. J., & Wolff, H. G. (1955). The night-eating syndrome: A pattern of food intake among certain obese patients. *American Journal of Medicine, 19*, 78–86.

Sugarman, H. J., Sugerman, E. L., DeMaria, E. J., Kellum, J. M., Kennedy, C., Mowery, Y., et al. (2003a). Bariatric surgery for severely obese adolescents.

Journal of Gastrointestinal Surgery, 7, 102–108.

Sugarman, H. J., Wolfe, L. G., Sica, D. A., & Clore, J. N. (2003b). Diabetes and hyptertension in severe obesity and effects of gastric bypass-induced weight loss. *Annals of Surgery, 237,* 751–756.

Sullivan, P. F. (1995). Mortality in anorexia nervosa. *American Journal of Psychiatry, 152,* 1073–1074.

Sullivan, P. F., Bulik, C. M., Fear, J. L., & Pickering, A. (1998). Outcome of anorexia nervosa: A case-control study. *American Journal of Psychiatry, 155,* 939–946.

Sysko, R., Walsh, B. T., & Fairburn, C. G. (2005). EDE-Q as a measure of change in patients with bulimia nervosa. *International Journal of Eating Disorders, 37,* 100–106.

Szmukler, G., Wykes, T., & Parkman, S. (1998). Care giving and the impact on carers of the community mental health service. *British Journal of Psychiatry, 173,* 399–403.

Tanofsky-Kraff, M., Morgan, C. M., Yanovski, S. Z., Marmarosh, C., Wilfley, D. E., & Yanovski, J. A. (2003). Comparison of assessments of children's eating-disordered behaviors by interview and questionnaire. *International Journal of Eating Disorders, 33,* 213–224.

Tanofsky-Kraff, M., & Yanovski, S. Z. (2004). Eating disorder or disordered eating? Non-normative eating patterns in obese individuals. *Obesity Research, 12,* 1361–1366.

Tchanturia, K., Anderluh, B., Morris, R. G., et al. (2004). Cognitive flexibility in anorexia and bulimia nervosa. *Journal of the International Neuropsychological Society, 10,* 513–520.

Teachman, B. A., & Brownell, K. D. (2001). Implicit anti-fat bias among health professionals: Is anyone immune? *International Journal of Obesity, 25,* 1525–1531.

Telch, C. F., Agras, W. S., & Linehan, M. (2001). Dialectical behavior therapy for binge eating disorder. *Journal of Consulting and Clinical Psychology, 69,* 1061–1065.

Telch, C. F., Agras, W. S., & Rossiter, E. M. (1988). Binge eating increases with increasing adiposity. *International Journal of Eating Disorders, 7,* 115–119.

Telch, C. F., Agras, W. S., Rossiter, E. M., Wilfley, D., & Kenardy, J. (1990). Group cognitive-behavioral treatment for the non-purging bulimic: An initial evaluation. *Journal of Consulting and Clinical Psychology, 58,* 629–635.

Thiels, C., Schmidt, U., Treasure, J., Garthe, R., & Troop, N. (1998). Guided self-change for bulimia nervosa incorporating use of a self-care manual. *American Journal of Psychiatry, 155,* 947–953.

Tobin, D. L., Griffing, A., & Griffing, S. (1997). An examination of subtype criteria for bulimia nervosa. *International Journal of Eating Disorders, 22,* 179–186.

Toubro, S., & Astrup, A. (1997). Randomised comparison of diets for maintaining obese subjects' weight after major weight loss: Ad lib, low fat, high carbohydrate diet v fixed energy intake. *British Journal of Psychiatry, 314,* 29–34.

Touyz, S. W., Beumont, P. J. V., & Dunn, S. M. (1987). Behavior therapy in the management of patients with anorexia nervosa: A lenient flexible approach. *Psychotherapy and Psychosomartics, 48,* 151–156.

Touyz, S. W., Beumont, P. J., Glaun, D., Phillips, T., & Crowie, I. (1984). A comparison of lenient and strict operant conditioning programmes in refeeding patients with anorexia nervosa. *British Journal of Psychiatry, 144,* 517–520.

Tozzi, F., & Bulik, C. M. (2003). Candidate genes in eating disorders. *Current Drug Targets – CNS and Neurological Disorders, 2,* 31–39.

Tozzi, F., Thornton, L. M., Klump, K. L., Fichter, M. M., Halmi, K. A., Kaplan, A. S., et al. (2005). Symptom fluctuation in eating disorders: Correlates of diagnostic crossover. *American Journal of Psychiatry, 162*, 732–740.

Treasure, J., Murphy, T., Szmukler, T., Todd, G., Gavan, K., & Joyce, J. (2001). The experience of caregiving for severe mental illness: A comparison between anorexia nervosa and psychosis. *Social Psychiatry and Psychiatric Epidemiology, 36*, 343–347.

Treasure, J., Schmidt, U., Troop, N., Tiller, J., Todd, G., & Turnbull, S. (1996). Sequential treatment for bulimia nervosa incorporating a self-care manual. *British Journal of Psychiatry, 168*, 94–98.

Troiano, R. P., & Flegal, K. M. (1999). Overweight prevalence among youth in the United States: Why so many different numbers? *International Journal of Obesity and Related Metabolic Disorders, 23*, S22–S27.

Tsai, A. G., & Wadden, T. A. (2005). Systematic review: An evaluation of major commercial weight loss programs in the United States. *Annals of Internal Medicine, 142*, 56–66.

Tuomilehto, J., Lindstrom J, Eriksson, J. G., Valle, T. T., Hamalainen, H., Ilanne-Parikka, P., et al. (2001). Prevention of type 2 diabetes mellitus by changes in lifestyle among subjects with impaired glucose tolerance. *New England Journal of Medicine, 3*, 1343–1350.

Turnbull, S., Ward, A., Treasure, J., Jick, H., & Derby, L. (1996). The demand for eating disorder care. An epidemiological study using the General Practice Research Database. *British Journal of Psychiatry, 169*, 705–712.

Turner, H., & Bryant-Waugh, R. (2004). Eating disorder not otherwise specified (EDNOS): Profiles of clients presenting at a community eating disorder service.

European Eating Disorders Review, 12, 18–26.

Vague, J. (1947). Sexual differentiation, a factor affecting the forms of obesity. *Presse Medicale, 30*, 339–340.

Vandereycken, W. (1984). Neuroleptics in the short-term treatment of anorexia nervosa. A double-blind placebo-controlled study with sulpiride. *British Journal of Psychiatry, 144*, 288–292.

Vandereycken, W. (2002). History of anorexia nervosa and bulimia nervosa. In C. G. Fairburn & K. D. Brownell (Eds.), *Comprehensive textbook of eating disorders and obesity* (pp. 151–154). New York: Guildford Press.

Vandereycken, W., & Van Deth, R. (1994). *From fasting saints to anorexia girls: The history of self-starvation*. New York: New York University Press.

Venables, J. F. (1930). Anorexia nervosa: A study of the pathogenesis and treatment of nine cases. *Guy's Hospital Report, 80*, 213–216.

von Ranson, K. M., Kaye, W. H., Weltzin, T. E., Rao, R., & Matsunaga, H. (1999). Obsessive-compulsive disorder symptoms before and after recovery from bulimia nervosa. *American Journal of Psychiatry, 156*, 1703–1708.

Wadden, T. A., Anderson, D. A., Foster, G. D., Bennett, A., Steinberg, C., & Sarwer, D. B. (2000). Obese women's perceptions of their physicians' weight management attitudes and practices. *Archives of Family Medicine, 9*, 854–860.

Wadden, T. A., Berkowitz, R. I., Sarwer, D. B., Prus-Wisniewski, R., & Steinberg, C. (2001). Benefits of lifestyle modification in the pharmacologic treatment of obesity: A randomized trial. *Archives of Internal Medicine, 161*, 218–227.

Wadden, T. A. Foster, G. D., & Letizia, K. A. (1992). Response of obese binge eaters to behavior therapy combined with very low calorie diet. *Journal of*

Consulting and Clinical Psychology, 60, 808–881.

Wadden, T. A., Foster, G. D., & Letizia, K. A. (1994). One-year behavioral treatment of obesity: Comparison of moderate and severe caloric restriction and the effects of weight maintenance therapy. *Journal of Consulting and Clinical Psychology, 62,* 165–171.

Wadden, T. A., Foster, G. D., Sarwer, D. B., Anderson, D. A., Gladis, M., Sanderson, R. S., et al. (2004). Dieting and the development of eating disorders in obese women: Results of a randomized controlled trial. *American Journal of Clinical Nutrition, 80,* 560–568.

Wadden, T. A., Steen, S. N., Wingate, B. J., & Foster, G. D. (1996). Psychosocial consequences of weight reduction: How much weight loss is enough? *American Journal of Clinical Nutrition, 63,* 461S–465S.

Wadden, T. A., Sternberg, J. A., Letizia, K. A., Stunkard, A. J., & Foster, G. D. (1989). Treatment of obesity by very low calorie diet, behavior therapy, and their combination: A five-year perspective. *International Journal of Obesity, 13,* 39–46.

Wadden, T. A., Stunkard, A. J., & Liebschutz, J. (1988). Three-year follow-up of the treatment of obesity by very low calorie diet, behavior therapy, and their combination. *Journal of Consulting and Clinical Psychology, 56,* 925–928.

Wadden, T. A., Van Itallie, T. B., & Blackburn, G. (1990). Responsible and irresponsible use of very-low-calorie-diets in the treatment of obesity. *Journal of American Medical Association, 263,* 83–85.

Wadden, T. A., Vogt, R. A., Andersen, R. E., Bartlett, S. J., Foster, G. D., Kuehnel, R. H., et al. (1997). Exercise in the treatment of obesity: Effects of four interventions on body composition, resting energy expenditure, appetite,
and mood. *Journal of Consulting and Clinical Psychology, 65,* 269–277.

Wadden, T. A., Womble, L. G., Sarwer, D. B., Berkowitz, R. I., Clark, V. L., & Foster, G. D. (2003). Great expectations: "I'm losing 25% of my weight no matter what you say". *Journal of Clinical and Consulting Psychology, 72,* 1084–1089.

Wade, T. D., Bulik, C. M., Neale, M., et al. (2000). Anorexia nervosa and major depression: Shared genetic and environmental risk factors. *American Journal of Psychiatry, 157,* 469–471.

Walsh, B. T., & Boudreau, G. (2003). Laboratory studies of binge eating disorder. *International Journal of Eating Disorders, 34,* S30–S38.

Walsh, B. T., & Cameron, V. L. (2005). *If your adolescent has an eating disorder.* New York: Oxford University Press.

Walsh, B. T., Fairburn, C. G., Mickley, D., Sysko, R., & Parides, M. K. (2004). Treatment of bulimia nervosa in a primary care setting. *American Journal of Psychiatry, 161,* 556–561.

Walsh, B. T., Hadigan, C. M., Devlin, M. J., Gladis, M., & Roose, S. P. (1991). Long-term outcome of antidepressant treatment for bulimia nervosa. *American Journal of Psychiatry, 148,* 1206–1212.

Walsh, B. T., Kaplan, A. S., Attia, E., Carter, J., Devlin, M. J., Olmsted, M., et al. (2005, September–October). *Fluoxetine versus placebo to prevent relapse in anorexia nervosa: Primary outcome of drug on time to relapse in 93 weight restored subjects.* Paper presented at the Eating Disorders Research Society 11th Annual Meeting, Toronto, Ontario.

Walsh, B. T., Kissileff, H.R, Cassidy, S. M., & Dantzic, S. (1989). Eating behavior of women with bulimia. *Archives of General Psychiatry, 46,* 54–58.

Walsh, B. T., Kissileff, H. R., & Hadigan, C. M. (1989). Eating behavior in bulimia. *Annals of the New York Academy of Sciences, 575,* 446–454.

Walsh, B. T., Wilson, G. T., Loeb, K. L., Devlin, M.J, Pike, K. M., Roose, S. P., et al. (1997). Medication and psychotherapy in the treatment of bulimia nervosa. *American Journal of Psychiatry, 154,* 523–531.

Wang, S. S., Brownell, K. D., & Wadden, T. A. (2004). The influence of the stigma of obesity on overweight individuals. *International Journal of Obesity and Metabolic Disorders, 28,* 1333–1337.

Wansink, B. (2004). Environmental factors that increase the food intake and consumption volume of unknowing consumers. *Annual Review of Nutrition, 24,* 455–479.

Wansink, B., & Cheney, M. M. (2005). Super bowls: Serving bowl size and food consumption. *Journal of the American Medical Association, 293,* 1727–1728.

Wansink, B., & Kim, J. (2005). Bad popcorn in big buckets: Portion size can influence intake as much as taste. *Journal of Nutrition Education Behavior, 37,* 242–245.

Wansink, B., Painter, J. E., & North, J. (2005). Bottomless bowls: Why visual cues of portion size may influence intake. *Obesity Research, 13,* 93–100.

Warheit, G. J., Langer, L. M., Zimmerman, R. S., & Biafora, F. A. (1993). Prevalence of bulimic behaviors and bulimia among a sample of the general population. *American Journal of Epidemiology, 137,* 569–576.

Watson, T. L., Bowers, W. A., & Anderson, A. E. (2000). Involuntary treatment of eating disorders. *American Journal of Psychiatry, 157,* 1806–1810.

Weaver, K., Wuest, J., & Ciliska, D. (2005). Understanding women's journey of recovering from anorexia nervosa. *Qualitative Health Research, 15,* 188–206.

Westenhoefer, J. (2001). Prevalence of eating disorders and weight control practices in Germany in 1990 and 1997. *International Journal of Eating Disorders, 29,* 477–481.

Whitaker, A., Johnson, J., Shaffer, D., Rapoport, J. L., Kalikow, K., Walsh, B. T., et al. (1990). Uncommon troubles in young people: Prevalence estimates of selected psychiatric disorders in a non-referred adolescent population. *Archives of General Psychiatry, 47,* 487–496.

White, M. A., & Grilo, C. M. (2006). Psychiatric comorbidity in binge eating disorder as a function of smoking history. *Journal of Clinical Psychiatry, 67,* 594–599.

Whittal, M. L., Agras, W. S., & Gould, R. A. (1999). Bulimia nervosa: A meta-analysis of psychosocial and pharmacological treatments. *Behavior Therapy, 30,* 117–135.

Wilfley, D. E., Agras, W. S., Telch, C. F., Rossiter E. M., Schneider, J. A., Cole, A. G., et al. (1993). Group cognitive-behavioral therapy and group interpersonal psychotherapy for the nonpurging bulimic individual: A controlled comparison. *Journal of Consulting and Clinical Psychology, 61,* 296–305.

Wilfley, D. E., Friedman, M. A., Dounchis, J. Z., Stein, R. I., Welch, R. R., & Ball, S. (2000a). Comorbid psychopathology in binge eating disorder: Relation to eating disorder severity at baseline and following treatment. *Journal of Consulting and Clinical Psychology, 68,* 641–649.

Wilfley, D. E., Grilo, C. M., & Rodin, J. (1997). Group psychotherapy for the treatment of bulimia nervosa and binge eating disorder: Research and clinical methods. In J. L. Spira (Ed.), *Group therapy for medically ill patients* (pp. 225–295). New York: Guilford Press.

Wilfley, D. E., MacKenzie, K. R., Welch, R. R., Ayes, V. E., & Weissman, M. M.

(2000). *Interpersonal psychotherapy for group*. New York: Basic Books.

Wilfley, D. E., Schwartz, M. B., Spurrell, E. B., & Fairburn, C. G. (2000b). Using the eating disorder examination to identify the specific psychopathology of binge eating disorder. *International Journal of Eating Disorders, 27*, 259–269.

Wilfley, D. E., Welch, R. R., Stein, R. I., Spurrell, E. B., Cohen, L. R., Saelens, B. E., et al. (2002). A randomized comparison of group cognitive-behavioral therapy and group interpersonal psychotherapy for the treatment of overweight individuals with binge eating disorder. *Archives of General Psychiatry, 59*, 713–721.

Wilfley, D. E., Wilson, G. T., & Agras, W. S. (2003). The clinical significance of binge eating disorder. *International Journal of Eating Disorders, 34*, S96–S106.

Willet, W. C. (1998). Dietary fat and obesity: An unconvincing relation. *American Journal of Clinical Nutrition, 68*, 1149–1150.

Williamson, D. A., Gleaves, D. H., & Stewart, T. M. (2005). Categorical versus dimensional models of eating disorders: An examination of the evidence. *International Journal of Eating Disorders, 37*, 1–10.

Williamson, D. A., Womble, L. G., Smeets M. A., Netemeyer, R. G., Thaw, J. M., Kutlesic, V., et al. (2002). Latent structure of eating disorder symptoms: A factor analytic and taxometric investigation. *American Journal of Psychiatry, 159*, 412–418.

Wilson, G. T. (1992). Diagnostic criteria for bulimia nervosa. *International Journal of Eating Disorders, 11*, 315–319.

Wilson, G. T. (1994). Behavioral treatment of obesity: Thirty years and counting. *Advances in Behavior Research and Therapy, 16*, 31–75.

Wilson, G. T. (2005). Psychological treatment of eating disorders. *Annual Review of Clinical Psychology, 1*, 439–465.

Wilson, G. T., & Eldredge, K. L. (1991). Frequency of binge eating in bulimic patients: Diagnostic validity. *International Journal of Eating Disorders, 10*, 557–561.

Wilson, G. T., & Fairburn, C. G. (1993). Cognitive treatments for eating disorders. *Journal of Consulting and Clinical Psychology, 61*, 261–269.

Wilson, G. T., & Fairburn, C. G. (2000). The treatment of binge eating disorder. *European Eating Disorders Review, 8*, 351–354.

Wilson, G. T., Fairburn, C. G., & Agras, W. S. (1997). Cognitive-behavioral therapy for bulimia nervosa. In D. M. Garner & P. E. Garfinkel (Eds.), *Handbook of treatment for eating disorders* (pp. 67–93). New York: Guilford Press.

Wilson, G. T., Fairburn, C. G., Agras, W. S., Walsh, B. T., & Kraemer, H. (2002). Cognitive behavioral therapy for bulimia nervosa: Time course and mechanisms of change. *Journal of Consulting and Clinical Psychology, 70*, 267–274.

Wilson, G. T., Loeb, K. L., Walsh, B. T., Labouvie, E., Petkova, E., Liu, X., et al. (1999). Psychological versus pharmacological treatments of bulimia nervosa: Predictors and process of change. *Journal of Consulting and Clinical Psychology, 67*, 451–459.

Wilson, G. T., & Shafran, R. (2005). Eating disorders guidelines from NICE. *Lancet, 365*, 79–81.

Wilson, G. T., & Vitousek, K. M. (1999). Self-monitoring in the assessment of eating disorders. *Psychological Assessment, 11*, 480–489.

Windauer, U., Lennerts, W., Talbot, P., Touyz, S. W., & Beumont, P. J. (1993). How well are "cured" anorexia nervosa patients? An investigation of 16 weight-recovered anorexic patients. *British Journal of Psychiatry, 163*, 195–200.

Wing, R. R. (1999). Physical activity in the

treatment of the adulthood overweight and obesity: Current evidence and research issues. *Medicine and Science in Sports and Exercise, 31,* S547–S552.

Wing, R. R., Koeske, R., Epstein, H. L., Nowalk, M., Gooding, W., & Becker, D. (1987). Long-term effects of modest weight loss in type II diabetic patients. *Archives of Internal Medicine, 147,* 1749–1753.

Winn, S., Perkins, S., Murray, J., Murphy, R., & Schmidt, U. (2004). A qualitative study of the experience of caring for a person with bulimia nervosa. Part 2: carers' needs and experiences of services and other support. *International Journal of Eating Disorders, 36,* 269–279.

Wirth, A., & Krause, J. (2001). Long-term weight loss with sibutramine: A randomized controlled trial. *Journal of the American Medical Association, 286,* 1331–1339.

Wittchen, H. U., Nelson, C. B., & Lachner, G. (1998). Prevalence of mental disorders and psychosocial impairments in adolescents and young girls. *Psychological Medicine, 28,* 109–126.

Wittgrove, A. C., & Clark, G. W. (2000). Laparoscopic gastric bypass, Roux-en-Y – 500 patients: Technique and results, with 3–60 month follow-up. *Obesity Surgery, 10,* 233–239.

Wolf, A. M., & Colditz, G. A. (1998). Current estimates of the economic cost of obesity in the United States. *Obesity Research, 6,* 97–106.

Wood, P. D., Stefanick, M. L., Williams, P. T., & Haskell, W. L. (1991). The effects on plasma lipoproteins of a prudent weight-reducing diet, with or without exercise, in overweight men and women. *New England Journal of Medicine, 325,* 461–466.

World Health Organization. (1992). *International Classification of Diseases* (10th rev.). Geneva: World Health Organization.

World Health Organization. (1998). *Obesity: Preventing and managing the global epidemic: Report of a WHO Consultation on Obesity* (WHO/NUT/ NCD/97.2). Geneva: World Health Organization.

Yancy, W. S., Jr., Olsen, M. K., Guyton, J. R., Bakst, R. P., & Westman, E. C. (2004). A low-carbohydrate, ketogenic diet versus a low-fat diet to treat obesity and hyperlipidemia: A randomized, controlled trial. *Annals of Internal Medicine, 140,* 769–777.

Yanovski, S. Z. (1993). Binge eating disorder: Current knowledge and future directions. *Obesity Research, 1,* 306–324.

Yanovski, S. Z. (2003). Binge eating disorder and obesity in 2003: Could treating an eating disorder have a positive effect on the obesity epidemic? *International Journal of Eating Disorders, 34S,* S117–S120.

Yanovski, S. Z., Gormally, J. F., Leser, M. S., Gwirtsman, H. E., & Yanovski, J. A. (1994). Binge eating disorder affects outcome of comprehensive very-low-calorie diet treatment. *Obesity Research, 2,* 205–212.

Yanovski, S. Z., Leet, M., Yanovski, J. A., Flood, M., Gold, P. W., Kissileff, H. R., et al. (1992). Food selection and intake of obese women with binge-eating disorder. *American Journal of Clinical Nutrition, 56,* 975–980.

Yanovski, S. Z., Nelson, J. E., Dubbert B. K., & Spitzer, R. L. (1993). Association of binge eating disorder and psychiatric comorbidity in obese subjects. *American Journal of Psychiatry, 150,* 1472–1479.

Zipfel, S., Lowe, B., Reas, D. L., Deter, H. C., & Herzog, W. (2000). Long-term prognosis in anorexia nervosa: Lessons from a 21-year follow-up study. *Lancet, 355,* 721–722.

Zipfel, S., Reas, D. L., Thornton, C., Olmsted, M. P., Williamson, D. A., Gerlinghoff, M., et al. (2002). Day hospitalization programs for eating disorders: A systematic review of the literature. *International Journal of Eating Disorders, 31,* 105–117.

Zuercher, J. N., Cumella, E. J., Woods, B. K., Eberly, M., & Carr, J. K. (2003). Efficacy of voluntary nasogastric tube feeding in female inpatients with anorexia nervosa. *JPEN Journal of Parenteral and Enteral Nutrition, 27,* 268–276.

Author index

Subject index

constipation 73
coronary heart disease, obesity and 149–50
culture-bound syndromes 37

depression 49, 53
  in anorexia nervosa 42, 76, 77
  in binge eating disorder 125
  in bulimia nervosa 100
  post-partum 75
  weight gain and 63
dermatological abnormalities in anorexia nervosa 73–4
desipramine, binge eating disorder 134
dexfenfluramine 170
diabetes
  gestational, obesity in children and 46
  type I 121–3, 124
  type II 24, 121–3, 148, 150–1, 178
Diagnostic and Statistical Manual of Mental Disorders (DSM-IV) 3
diagnostic schemes 2–3
dialectical behavior therapy (DBT), in binge eating disorder 133
diet pills 13, 33, 35
dietary fat intake 55
diethylpropion 170
dietin resistance 164
dieting 35–6
  in anorexia nervosa 80–1
  in binge eating disorder 129–30
  obesity 163–4
  prevalence 31–2
disgust, feelings of 20
disordered eating versus eating disorders 24–5
distribution of eating disorders 27–8, 36–7
diuretics 5, 13, 15, 33, 35, 36
dumping syndrome 182
duodenal switch procedure 177
dyslipidemia, obesity and 150, 152

Eating Disorder Examination (EDE) 71–2

Eating Disorder Not Otherwise Specified (EDNOS) 3, 15–17, 27
  assessment 119–21
  assessment instruments 120–1
  current guidelines 127–9
  development and course 44–5
  future treatment directions 127–9
  pharmacotherapy 127
  prevalence 28
  recovery rate 78
  transdiagnostic model for assessment/ treatment 128
  treatment needs 126–7
Eating Disorders Examination – Questionnaire Version (EDE-Q) 72, 98, 126
eating related concerns, prevalence 30–1
  increase in 35–6
embarrassment 12, 120
enemas, misuse of 13, 15
environmental risk factors 46–7, 49, 53
epidemiology of eating disorders 27–8
ethnic minority groups 37, 38, 39
evening hyperphagia (overeating) 25
exercise, excessive 5, 7, 13, 14, 15
  obesity and 60–2, 167–9

familial liability 49–51
familial obesity 53
family therapy 82–5
fast food 59–60
fasting 13
Fasting Plasma Glucose Test (FPG) 123
fear of fat 5, 8
Feeding Disorder of Infancy or Early Childhood 3
fenfluramine 170
fluoxetine 109, 116–17
  in anorexia nervosa 86–7
  in binge eating disorder 138–9
  in bulimia nervosa 102
Food Guide Pyramid 162–3, 175
frustration in clinicians 89

gallbladder disease, obesity and 152
gallstones, obesity and 152
gastric banding 176, 178

Take off Pounds Sensibly 158
Therapeutic Contract Program (TCP)
   128–9
topiramate, binge eating disorder and 132

upper-body (android-type) obesity 23–4,
   147–8

vertical banded gastroplasty 176
very-low-calorie diets (VLCD) 160, 164–5

vomiting 33, 35, 120
   self-induced 5, 13–14, 36
voracity 2

weight control, prevalence 31–3
weight related concerns, prevalence 30–1,
   35–6
Weight Watchers 158, 159

Zone diet 159